SWEET & SAVORY
KETO CHAFFLES

75
Delicious Treats
for Your Low-Carb Diet

Martina Slajerova
Best-selling author of
The KetoDiet Cookbook

FAIR WINDS

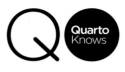

Inspiring | Educating | Creating | Entertaining

Brimming with creative inspiration, how-to projects, and useful information to enrich your everyday life, Quarto Knows is a favorite destination for those pursuing their interests and passions. Visit our site and dig deeper with our books into your area of interest: Quarto Creates, Quarto Cooks, Quarto Homes, Quarto Lives, Quarto Drives, Quarto Explores, Quarto Gifts, or Quarto Kids.

First Published in 2020 by Fair Winds Press, an imprint of The Quarto Group,
100 Cummings Center, Suite 265-D, Beverly, MA 01915, USA.
T (978) 282-9590 F (978) 283-2742 QuartoKnows.com

Fair Winds Press titles are also available at discount for retail, wholesale, promotional, and bulk purchase. For details, contact the Special Sales Manager by email at specialsales@quarto.com or by mail at The Quarto Group, Attn: Special Sales Manager, 100 Cummings Center, Suite 265-D, Beverly, MA 01915, USA.

24 23 22 21 20   2 3 4 5

ISBN: 978-1-59233-972-3

Digital edition published in 2020
eISBN: 978-1-63159-915-6

Library of Congress Cataloging-in-Publication Data

Names: Slajerova, Martina, author.
Title: Sweet & savory keto chaffles : 75 delicious treats for your low-carb
    diet / Martina Slajerova.
Other titles: Sweet and savory keto chaffles
Description: Beverly, MA : Fair Winds Press, 2020.
Identifiers: LCCN 2020010700 (print) | LCCN 2020010701 (ebook) | ISBN
    9781592339723 (trade paperback) | ISBN 9781631599156 (ebook)
Subjects: LCSH: Pancakes, waffles, etc. | Low-carbohydrate diet--Recipes. |
    LCGFT: Cookbooks.
Classification: LCC TX770.P34 S56 2020 (print) | LCC TX770.P34 (ebook) |
    DDC 641.5/638--dc23
LC record available at https://lccn.loc.gov/2020010700
LC ebook record available at https://lccn.loc.gov/2020010701

Cover Image: Martina Slajerova
Page Layout: Megan Jones Design
Photography and Styling: Martina Slajerova
and Jo Harding modernfoodstories.com

Printed in China

The information in this book is for educational purposes only. It is not intended to replace the advice of a physician or medical practitioner. Please see your health-care provider before beginning any new health program.

I would like to thank my good friend Jo Harding, an awesome photographer and foodie without whom this book would have never become a reality.

To my soulmate Nikos, and to my mum and dad, who have always supported me, encouraged me, and believed in me. I can't thank you enough for everything you have done for me.

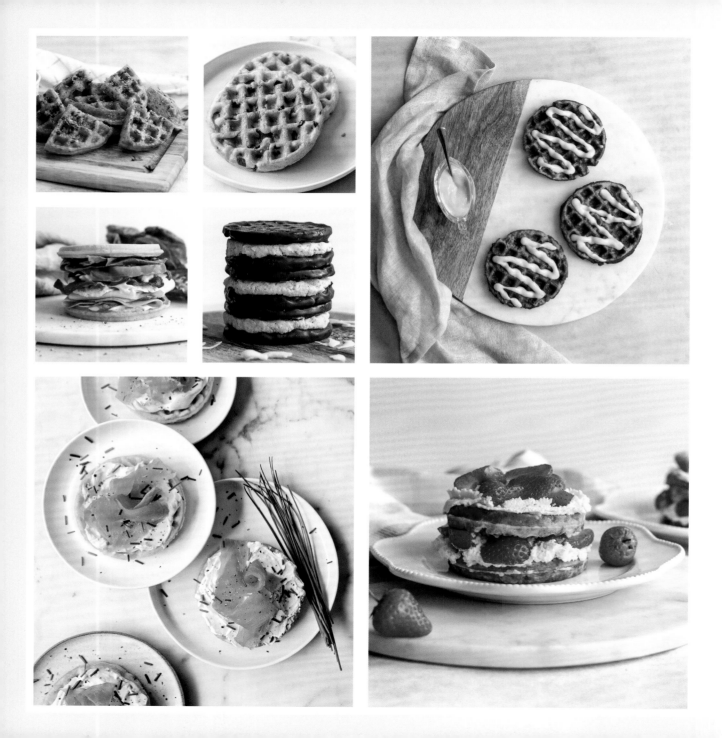

Contents

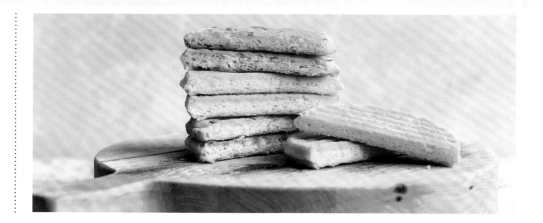

Chapter 1

Why Chaffles?

Chaffles—cheese waffles—are the new trend in the low-carb and keto community, and they have taken over on social media. That's for good reason: Chaffles are super fuss-free and versatile, and you only need a few common ingredients to make them. They can be used to make bread, sandwiches, or even a slice of cake!

How to Make Chaffles

The basic chaffle is made with just two ingredients: cheese and eggs. Although I love the simplicity, the texture is soft, cheesy, and eggy, which is not necessarily what you desire. I've tried and tested every possible way there is to make these wonderful keto waffles to bring you 75 creative recipes with the best textures and flavors. Apart from the chaffle recipes, I will show you how to swap individual ingredients to make them dairy-free, nut-free, and even egg-free.

MINI WAFFLE MAKER VERSUS REGULAR WAFFLE MAKER

To make mini chaffles, you'll need a 4-inch (10-cm) Dash Mini Waffle Maker. You can find one for around $15. In addition to the waffle grid, you can even get a mini panini maker from the same brand; it can be used interchangeably. Don't worry if you don't have a mini waffle maker; you can use a regular-sized waffle maker. If you do that, the yield will change and instead of 2 to 3 small round chaffles, you'll get 1½ to 2 regular-sized (5-inch/12.5-cm) Belgian square chaffles, or 1 to 1¼ large (7-inch/18-cm) round Belgian waffles. Chaffles made in a Belgian waffle maker tend to be drier and may crisp up more, so keep that in mind. If you don't have a waffle maker, simply cook the batter on a greased pan just like pancakes!

THE BEST CHEESE FOR CHAFFLES

Shredded part-skim, low-moisture mozzarella is ideal for both sweet and savory chaffles. For savory chaffles you can use any hard cheese, including mild or mature cheddar, Monterey Jack, Swiss cheese, Emmental, goat or sheep cheese, or the like. If you can't eat dairy, some types of grated hard vegan cheese will work. The ones I've tested were coconut- and almond-based. Keep in mind that not all vegan cheeses are healthy (always check the label) and most are relatively high in carbs. If you can't use cheese, you can always make Classic Keto Waffles without it. To do that, simply mix all of the ingredients and follow the steps for Basic Chaffles (page 14).

THE BEST SWEETENERS FOR CHAFFLES

To keep your chaffles low in carbs, use natural low-carb sweeteners such as erythritol, Swerve (made with erythritol and inulin), monk fruit, and stevia. Keep in mind swapping granulated sweeteners for stevia will affect the yield, as stevia does not have bulking effects. You can also use xylitol and yacon syrup in moderation.

Allulose is used in some recipes, such as keto-friendly caramel treats (Keto Caramel, page 11) and other desserts such as marshmallows (see page 140 for S'mores Chaffles). The carb count in allulose is similar to erythriol and the calories are similar to xylitol. It's as sweet as sugar and, just like sugar, it has the ability to caramelize. Unlike erythritol, it does not crystalize, and it is a great option in chilled desserts. If you can't find allulose, swap it for a powdered erythritol-based sweetener such as Swerve. The results won't be as smooth, but it is a good alternative.

BLENDING VERSUS MIXING

You can simply mix the batter using a fork or a whisk. For best results I always recommend blending the batter, especially if you're making sweet chaffles. It's worth the extra effort as it makes chaffles fluffier, improves the texture, and masks any eggy taste. Also, blending makes the batter thick and reduces the risk of it spilling over the waffle maker while it's cooking.

If you're using sweeteners, it's better to stir them in *after* the blending. Adding the sweetener before blending makes the batter a little runnier and more likely to leak out of the waffle maker. The blender you use will determine how smooth the batter is and may affect the number of chaffles you get. Any small blender, small food processor, or immersion blender will work. Blending is easier for large batches of chaffle batter.

Classic Keto Waffles

6 tablespoons (48 g/1.7 oz) almond flour or 2 tablespoons (16 g/0.6 oz) coconut flour

2 tablespoons (12 g/0.4 oz) whey protein powder or egg white protein powder

1 large egg

3 tablespoons (45 ml) unsweetened almond milk

1 tablespoon (15 ml) melted ghee, butter, or coconut oil

¼ teaspoon gluten-free baking powder

Pinch of salt and pepper for savory waffles OR 2 to 4 tablespoons granulated low-carb sweetener for sweet waffles

NOTE:

✱ For crispier waffles, use a few tablespoons more almond flour (do not substitute with coconut flour).

HOW TO STORE CHAFFLES

Cooked chaffles can be stored for up to 3 days at room temperature or in the fridge for up to 1 week. Wrapping the chaffles in aluminum foil keeps them fresh. Zip-top-bags, however, make them sweat and they can go moldy. Cooked chaffles can be frozen for up to 3 months and allowed to defrost at room temperature. To reheat chaffles, pop them in a toaster, waffle maker, or oven for a few minutes to crisp up.

WHAT TEXTURE SHOULD I EXPECT?

Warm chaffles fresh from the waffle maker will be soft, and some types of sweet chaffles may be fragile. That's why it's best to first open the lid of your waffle maker and let the chaffle cool slightly for 15 to 30 seconds before using a spatula to gently transfer it to a cooling rack. As the chaffles cool down, they will harden and crisp up. Depending on the batter and the cheese you used, you'll get slightly different textures.

The cooking time for chaffles varies between 2 and 5 minutes, or even longer if you prefer your chaffles crispier. Be aware that some types of cheese, such as shredded mozzarella, and ingredients such as cacao powder and chocolate chips may burn. Make sure to check the chaffles after 2 minutes and then after every 1 minute until they're ready.

HOW MANY CHAFFLES PER PERSON?

Most recipes in this book make 2 savory or 3 sweet chaffles. Depending on the occasion and type of meal, you can serve 1 to 2 chaffles per person. I made it easy; most recipes list values per individual chaffle.

LEAKPROOF TIPS TO ENSURE YOUR CHAFFLES DON'T OVERFLOW

The size of the egg matters. A large egg should weigh approximately 50 grams (1.8 oz), and a large egg white will weigh about 33 g/1.2 oz, but you may get 10–20% more or less even if it's a "large" egg. The recipe will still work with a slightly larger egg, but the batter is more likely to leak out of your waffle maker.

With a mini waffle maker, you will be working with small amounts of batter and there will be a risk of it overflowing. Always keep an eye on the batter. If it's about to overflow, slightly lift the lid to reduce the pressure on the batter. This should stop the leak. You can also use a spatula to gently move any batter that is about to leak out back inside.

Another way to prevent leaking is to add the batter in two parts per chaffle. To do that, spoon part of the batter into the waffle maker. Close the lid and cook for 1 minute. Lift the lid and spoon more batter in. Close the lid and cook for 2 to 4 minutes.

Make sure to stick with the recommended amount of baking powder. You'll need less baking powder for sweet chaffles than you will for savory chaffles, as most sweeteners also act as a raising agent. If you use too much baking powder, the batter is more likely to overflow and your chaffle maker will get messy.

If you can't find gluten-free baking powder, use a combination of baking soda and cream of tartar. For every 1 teaspoon baking powder, use ½ teaspoon cream of tartar plus ¼ teaspoon of baking soda (best mixed in advance or used in large batches). Instead of cream of tartar, you can use the same amount of another acidic ingredient, such as apple cider vinegar or lemon juice, added directly to the batter. Finally, never put the baking powder on top when blending, as some of it may get stuck to the lid and affect the yield.

ADJUSTING MACROS IN CHAFFLES

Some of the recipes are quite high in calories, especially some of the burgers and sandwiches. If you practice intermittent fasting and often skip a meal like I do, they are ideal for you. If you prefer more smaller meals instead, you may need to eat just half a serving. That's why in most recipes I list values per ½ sandwich or 1 chaffle, so you can easily double the serving size if you want to.

Any chaffle toppings and the cheese you use to make your chaffles will also make a difference to the macronutrient values. Most types of cheese are very low in carbs, although the values differ (e.g., 3.2 g net carbs per ½ cup grated part-skim low-moisture mozzarella but only 1.7 g net carbs per ½ cup grated cheddar). Different types of cheese will also contain different amount of fat and protein (e.g., cheddar contains more fat and calories and less protein than mozzarella), and you can use them to adjust the recipes. All sweet chaffles in this book use mozzarella cheese. Unless stated otherwise, all Basic Savory Chaffles (page 14) use cheddar.

ALLERGY SWAPS

By following the swaps below and those listed on page 15, you can adjust almost any chaffles to any dietary needs.

* Heavy whipping cream or mascarpone **>** coconut cream

* Almond milk **>** coconut milk or seed milk

* Nuts and nut butters **>** seeds, seed butters, and coconut butter

* Butter in sweet chaffles **>** palm shortening (use sustainable sources)

* Butter for cooking **>** ghee, duck fat, lard, or even olive oil (only light cooking)

How to Use This Book

Nutrition values for each recipe in this book are per serving unless stated otherwise. The nutrition data are derived from the USDA National Nutrient Database (ndb.nal.usda.gov).

Nutrition facts are calculated from edible parts. For example, if one large avocado is listed as 200 g/ 7.1 oz, this value represents its edible parts (pit and peel removed) unless otherwise specified.

Optional ingredients and suggested sides and toppings are not included in the nutrition information.

You can use raw cacao powder and unsweetened cocoa powder (Dutch process) interchangeably. Ingredients are all full-fat unless otherwise specified. All ingredients should be sugar-free, unless you use dark 85% to 90% chocolate, which contains a small and acceptable amount of sugar.

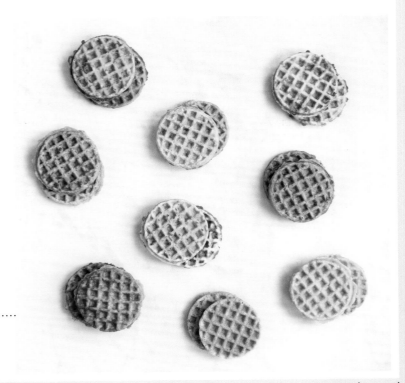

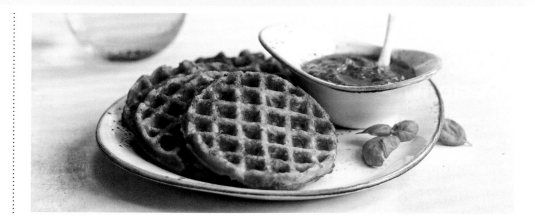

Chapter 2

Basics

Marinara Sauce

(makes about 1¼ cups/300 ml)

To make a medium jar of marinara sauce (300 g/10.5 oz), you'll need: 1 cup (150 g/5.3 oz) cherry tomatoes; ½ to 1 cup (8 to 15 g/0.3 to 0.5 oz) fresh basil; 2 cloves garlic; 1 small (30 g/1.1 oz) shallot or onion of choice; ¼ cup (60 g/2.2 oz) tomato purée; ¼ cup (60 ml) extra-virgin olive oil; ¼ teaspoon salt; and freshly ground pepper to taste.

   Place all the ingredients in a food processor and blend until smooth. When done, place in a sealed container and store in the fridge for up to 1 week.

Pesto Two Ways

(each makes about 1 cup/240 ml)

To make green pesto, you'll need: 2 cups (30 g/ 1.1 oz) fresh basil or herbs of choice (parsley, cilantro, and mint work best); ⅓ cup (45 g/ 1.6 oz) macadamia nuts, blanched almonds, or hulled sunflower seeds; 2 tablespoons (15 g/0.5 oz) pine nuts or more sunflower seeds; 4 cloves garlic, minced; 1 teaspoon fresh lemon zest; 1 tablespoon (15 ml) fresh lemon juice; ½ cup (120 ml) extra-virgin olive oil; sea salt; and black pepper. Optionally, you can add ⅓ cup (30 g/1.1 oz) grated Parmesan cheese and/or 4 to 6 pieces of drained sun-dried tomatoes.

Place all the ingredients in a blender. Process until smooth, and then season with sea salt and black pepper to taste.

To make red pesto, you'll need: 4 pitted olives (12 g/0.4 oz); ¼ cup (34 g/1.2 oz) macadamia nuts; 1 tablespoon (10 g/0.4 oz) pine nuts; ½ cup (55 g/1.9 oz) drained sun-dried tomatoes; 3 cloves garlic, peeled and sliced; ½ tablespoon fresh lemon juice or apple cider vinegar; 2 tablespoons (30 ml) unsweetened tomato paste; 1 cup (15 g/0.5 oz) fresh basil leaves; ¼ cup (60 ml) extra-virgin olive oil; and a pinch of fine sea salt and black pepper. Optionally, you can add ¼ cup (23 g/ 0.8 oz) grated Parmesan cheese.

Place all of the ingredients in a food processor and pulse until smooth.

You can keep your pesto in the fridge for up to 1 to 2 weeks. Always remember to add a thin layer of olive oil on top before you place it back in the fridge. Or spoon it into an ice cube tray and place in the freezer. Once frozen, empty the tray into a resealable plastic bag. Keep your frozen pesto for up to 6 months.

Keto Caramel

(makes about 200 g/7 oz thick caramel, or about 1 cup/240 ml caramel sauce)

To make keto caramel, you'll need: ¼ cup (57 g/2 oz) unsalted butter; ½ cup (100 g/ 3.5 oz) granulated allulose (page 7); ½ cup (120 ml) heavy whipping cream; and a pinch of salt (optional).

Fill a bowl with ice water and set it aside. You will need this later to chill the caramel, so make sure the saucepan can fit without any water getting inside the saucepan.

Place butter and allulose in a saucepan and melt over medium-low heat. Once the butter has melted, the mixture will start to foam. Stir frequently with a rubber spatula or a balloon whisk.

Cook for about 5 minutes and then pour in whipping cream. Optionally, add a pinch of salt for salted caramel. Stir until well combined. Keep cooking for 10 to 15 minutes. (For runny sauce you'll only need to cook it for 5 minutes, but for thick caramel topping it will take up to 15 minutes.)

The caramel can burn easily as it thickens. Make sure to keep an eye on it and keep stirring.

When the caramel reaches your desired consistency, take the saucepan off the heat and place it in the ice water to cool. This will stop the cooking process and help the caramel thicken. Keep stirring until the caramel is close to room temperature. It will thicken more as it cools down.

Transfer the caramel to a jar and refrigerate for 30 to 60 minutes. You can store it in a sealed jar for up to 2 weeks.

NOTE:

✱ Allulose may not be easy to find. Sweeteners such as erythritol or Swerve can be used, but the caramel sauce won't be as smooth and may be a bit gritty.

Chapter 3

Savory Chaffles

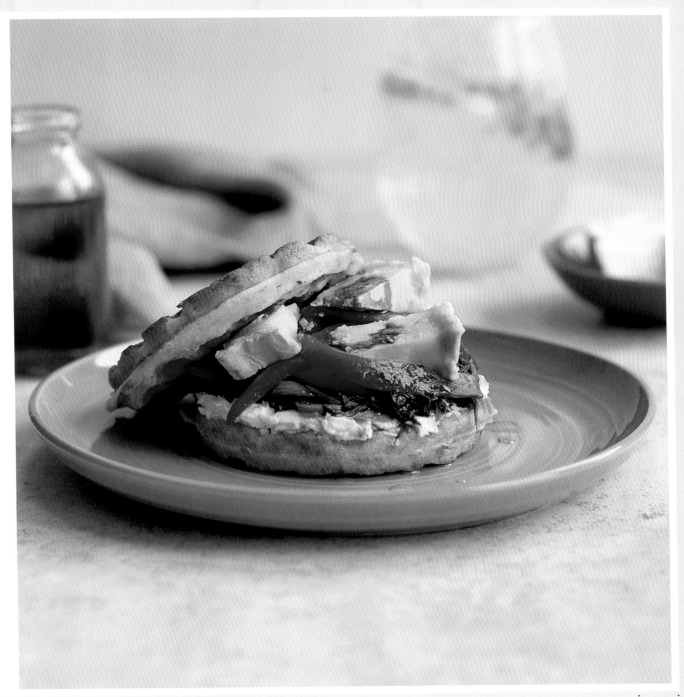

Servings:
2 mini savory chaffles / 3 sweet chaffles

Hands-on time:
5 minutes

Overall time:
10 minutes

Basic Chaffles Two Ways

This is the ultimate chaffle recipe fine-tuned to perfection. These chaffles go great with any sweet or savory filling or topping, or even served on their own as a side.

INGREDIENTS

Savory Chaffles

1 large egg

½ cup (57 g/2 oz) grated cheddar, mozzarella, or hard cheese of choice (see page 7 for tips)

¼ cup (25 g/0.9 oz) almond flour

¼ teaspoon gluten-free baking powder

Sweet Chaffles

1 large egg

½ cup (57 g/2 oz) grated mozzarella

¼ cup (25 g/0.9 oz) almond flour

⅛ teaspoon gluten-free baking powder

3 tablespoons (30 g/1.1 oz) granulated low-carb sweetener such as erythritol or Swerve, or to taste

Optional: ¼ to ½ teaspoon sugar-free vanilla extract, pinch of vanilla powder, or pinch of cinnamon

INSTRUCTIONS

Preheat the mini waffle maker (or read tips for regular-sized Belgian waffle makers on page 6). You can either place all of the ingredients in a bowl and mix until combined or process them in a blender or a food processor. A small capacity blender or an immersion blender with a tight fitting cup is ideal for blending small amounts of batter. Blending is optional but highly recommended. Blend the egg, cheese, almond flour, and baking powder.

For savory chaffles: To make 2 small savory waffles, spoon one-half of the batter (about 66 g/2.3 oz) into the hot waffle maker. Close the waffle maker and cook for 3 to 4 minutes. Repeat for the second waffle.

For sweet chaffles: Stir in the sweetener and vanilla or cinnamon (if using). Note: If you adjust the amount of sweetener, it may affect the yield. To make 3 small sweet waffles, spoon one-third of the batter (about 55 g/1.9 oz) into the hot waffle maker. Sweet chaffles tend to spread more than savory ones, so add them to the center as it spreads. Close the waffle maker and cook for 2 to 4 minutes,

Nutrition facts (1 savory chaffle/1 sweet chaffle)

Total carbs:	Fiber:	Net carbs:	Protein:	Fat:	Calories:	Calories from
3.5/3.3 g	1.2/0.8 g	2.3/2.4 g	12.3/8.3 g	18.4/9.7 g	224/131 kcal	carbs (4/7%) protein (22/26%) fat (74/67%)

checking the waffles after 2 minutes. Keep an eye on the batter in case it overflows (see leakproof tips on page 8). When done, open the lid and let cool down for 15 to 30 seconds. The chaffle will firm up as it cools. Use a spatula to gently transfer the chaffle onto a cooling rack. Repeat for the remaining batter.

The chaffles will be soft when they are warm, but they will crisp up as they cool down completely. Serve or store in a sealed container at room temperature for up to 3 days, or in the fridge for up to 1 week. The container will keep them soft, but you can leave them uncovered if you prefer them crispy.

NOTES

Depending on the preferred sweetness, you can use 2 to 4 tablespoons (20 to 40 g/0.7 to 1.4 oz) of granulated low-carb sweetener such as erythritol, Swerve, or even brown sugar substitute.

Nut-free Chaffles
Swap the ¼ cup (25 g/0.9 oz) almond flour for 1 tablespoon (8 g/0.3 oz) coconut flour OR 2 tablespoons (12 g/0.4 oz) fine sesame flour OR ¼ cup (25 g/0.9 oz) ground sunflower seeds OR 2½ tablespoons (18 g/0.6 oz) flax meal.

Egg-free Chaffles
Swap the egg for 1 tablespoon (7 g/0.3 oz) flax meal OR ground chia seeds, PLUS 3 tablespoons (45 ml) water. The texture will be crispier and less fluffy than chaffles made with eggs.

Dairy-free Chaffles
Swap ½ cup (57 g/2 oz) grated mozzarella for ½ cup (57 g/2 oz) grated vegan cheese. There are plenty of soy-free cheese alternatives made with coconut or nuts, but beware of the extra carbs.

Vegan Chaffles
To make chaffles that are both dairy-free and egg-free, swap the egg for 1 tablespoon (7 g/0.3 oz) flax meal OR ground chia seeds, PLUS 3 tablespoons (45 ml) water, and use ½ cup (57 g/ 2 oz) grated vegan cheese instead of the regular dairy cheese.

Eggy Taste? Not Crispy Enough? Try Egg White Chaffles.
Egg whites are ideal for creating a completely plain flavor with no eggy taste and a crispier result. To do that, swap the egg for 1 jumbo egg white or 2 small egg whites to get similar volume, or simply use 1 large egg white (slightly less volume).

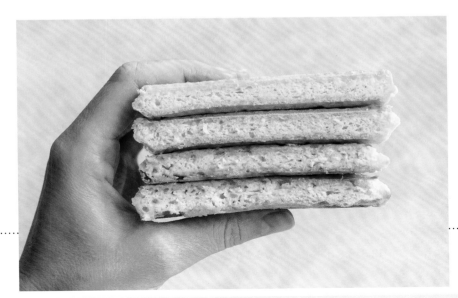

Everything Bagel Chaffles

These chaffles make the perfect base for sandwiches and bread options to serve with salads and dips. You can use ready-made seasoning or make your own— it's really easy! Here's a healthy way to enjoy all your favorite bagels with none of the carbs.

INGREDIENTS

Ingredients for 2 Basic Savory Chaffles (page 14)

1 tablespoon (14 g/0.5 oz) Everything Bagel Seasoning (see tip)

INSTRUCTIONS

Prepare a batch of the Basic Savory Chaffles by following the instructions on page 14. If you are using the blending method, add 2 teaspoons (9 g) of the bagel seasoning after the blending process and stir in. Sprinkle the remaining seasoning on top of the batter before closing the lid (½ teaspoon per chaffle). Store just like Basic Chaffles (page 8).

TIP

✱ To make your own "everything bagel seasoning," simply mix: 1 tablespoon (9 g/0.3 oz) white sesame seeds, 1 tablespoon (9 g/0.3 oz) black sesame seeds, 1½ tablespoons (13 g/0.4 oz) poppy seeds, 1 tablespoon (5 g/0.2 oz) dried minced onion (or 1 teaspoon onion powder), 1 tablespoon (3 g/ 0.1 oz) dried minced garlic (or 1 teaspoon garlic powder), and 1 teaspoon flaked or coarse sea salt. This will yield about ¼ cup (42 g/1.5 oz) of seasoning.

Nutrition facts (1 chaffle + topping)

Total carbs:	Fiber:	Net carbs:	Protein:	Fat:	Calories:	Calories from
5.9 g	**2.1 g**	**3.8 g**	**13.4 g**	**20.8 g**	**257 kcal**	**carbs (6%) protein (21%) fat (73%)**

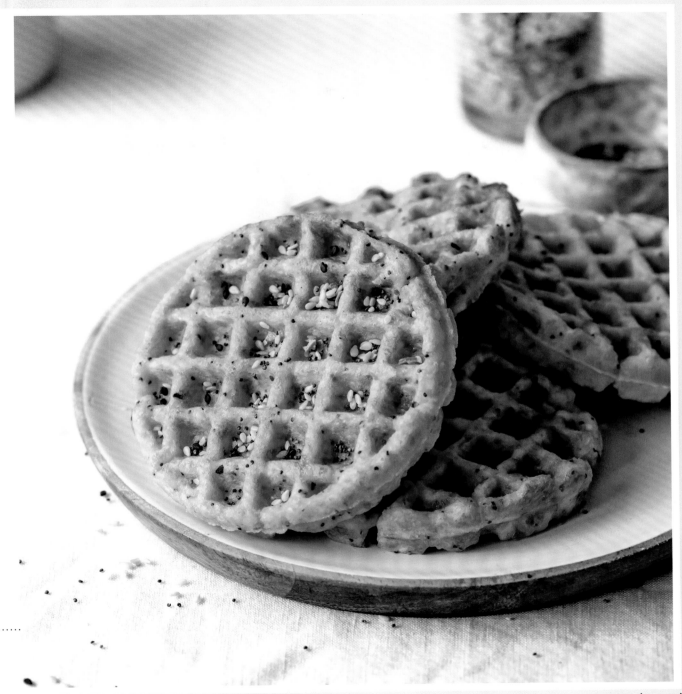

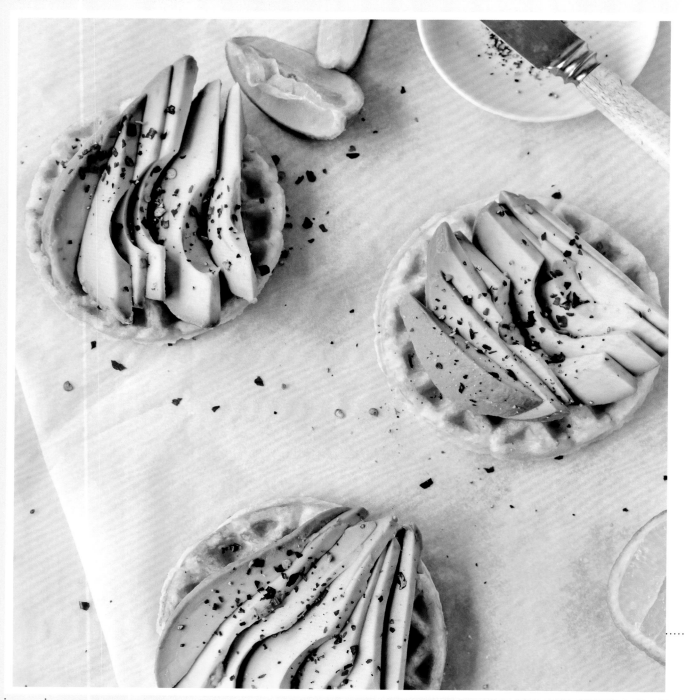

Servings:
2 mini chaffles

Hands-on time:
5 minutes

Overall time:
10 minutes

Avocado Toast Chaffles

This chaffle avocado toast is a delicious and simple breakfast, snack, or light meal. Feel free to use mashed instead of sliced avocado and add herbs, chopped onion, or garlic for a flavor boost.

INGREDIENTS

Ingredients for 2 Basic Savory Chaffles (page 14)

½ large (100 g/3.5 oz) avocado, peeled, pitted, and sliced

Pinch each of salt, black pepper, and red pepper flakes

INSTRUCTIONS

Prepare a batch of the Basic Savory Chaffles by following the instructions on page 14. Let the chaffles cool down and top with avocado. Sprinkle with salt, black pepper, and red pepper flakes. Serve immediately.

Nutrition facts (1 chaffle)

Total carbs:	Fiber:	Net carbs:	Protein:	Fat:	Calories:	Calories from
8 g	**4.7 g**	**3.3 g**	**13.3 g**	**25.8 g**	**306 kcal**	**carbs (4%) protein (18%) fat (78%)**

Rye Bread Chaffles

When I first gave up grains, I never missed sweets. What I missed most was a warm slice of rustic-style bread. This rye bread chaffle is incredibly satisfying and so good. Plus it's the fastest way to make keto bread. No more bread cravings!

INGREDIENTS

1 large egg white

½ cup (57 g/2 oz) grated mozzarella or other hard cheese

1 teaspoon toasted sesame oil

4 tablespoons (28 g/1 oz) flax meal

¼ teaspoon gluten-free baking powder

¼ teaspoon caraway seeds

Pinch each of salt and pepper

INSTRUCTIONS

Preheat the waffle maker. Blend the egg white, mozzarella, sesame oil, and 1 tablespoon (15 ml) water until smooth. Add the dry ingredients and blend again.

To cook the batter, follow the instructions for the Basic Savory Chaffles on page 14. When filling the waffle maker, use half (about 70 g/2.5 oz) of the batter for each chaffle. The batter will get thicker than your usual Basic Chaffles and is unlikely to leak, but keep an eye on it (see leakproof tips on page 8). Let the chaffles cool down and serve. They can be stored just like Basic Chaffles (page 8).

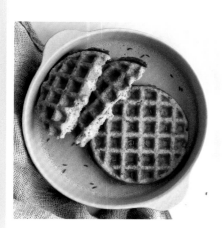

Nutrition facts (1 chaffle)

Total carbs:	Fiber:	Net carbs:	Protein:	Fat:	Calories:	Calories from
6 g	**3.9 g**	**2.1 g**	**11.1 g**	**13.8 g**	**188 kcal**	**carbs (5%)** **protein (25%)** **fat (70%)**

Salmon & Cream Cheese Chaffles

Who said healthy food cannot be tasty? These smoked salmon and cream cheese chaffles are ideal for breakfast, lunchboxes, and snacking. Start your day with a meal fueled with healthy fats and protein!

INGREDIENTS

Ingredients for 2 Basic Savory Chaffles (page 14)

¼ cup (60 g/2.1 oz) cream cheese

2–3 slices (57 g/2 oz) smoked salmon

1 tablespoon (3 g/0.1 oz) chopped chives or spring onion

Pinch of black pepper

INSTRUCTIONS

Prepare a batch of the Basic Savory Chaffles by following the instructions on page 14. Let the chaffles cool down and top with cream cheese (2 tablespoons per chaffle) and smoked salmon (1 oz/28 g per chaffle). Sprinkle with chives and black pepper and serve immediately.

TIP

* Swap the Basic Chaffles for Everything Bagel Chaffles on page 16.

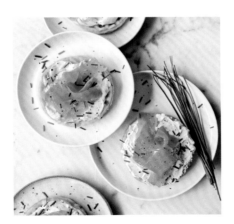

Nutrition facts (1 chaffle + topping)

Total carbs:	Fiber:	Net carbs:	Protein:	Fat:	Calories:	Calories from
4.6 g	**1.3 g**	**3.3 g**	**19.6 g**	**28 g**	**331 kcal**	**carbs (4%) protein (23%) fat (73%)**

Servings:
2 mini chaffles

Hands-on time:
10 minutes

Overall time:
15 minutes

Jalapeño Popper Chaffles

Do you like jalapeño poppers? Then you'll love these spicy Mexican-style chaffles! Eat them on their own or use them just like bread to make a sandwich packed with heat and flavor.

INGREDIENTS

2 thin-cut slices (30 g/1.1 oz) of bacon, chopped

1 large egg

½ cup (57 g/2 oz) grated cheddar or other hard cheese

¼ cup (25 g/0.9 oz) almond flour

¼ teaspoon gluten-free baking powder

1 small (14 g/0.5 oz) jalapeño pepper, sliced or chopped and seeds removed

INSTRUCTIONS

Start by crisping up the bacon pieces. To do that, put the bacon in a hot pan and add a tablespoon (15 ml) of water. Cook over medium-low heat until the bacon grease is rendered and cook for 1 to 2 more minutes to crisp up. Then take it off the heat.

Follow the instructions for the Basic Savory Chaffles on page 14. If you are using the blending method, add the crisp bacon (excluding excess bacon grease) and jalapeño pepper after the blending process and stir in. They can be stored just like Basic Chaffles (page 8).

Nutrition facts (1 chaffle)

Total carbs:	Fiber:	Net carbs:	Protein:	Fat:	Calories:	Calories from
4 g	**1.5 g**	**2.5 g**	**14.7 g**	**19.2 g**	**243 kcal**	**carbs (4%)** **protein (24%)** **fat (72%)**

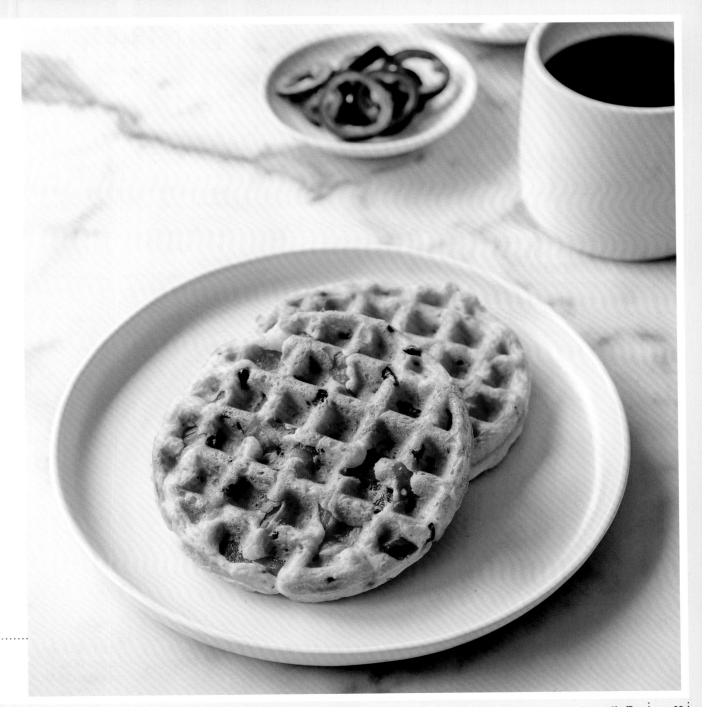

Servings:
2 mini chaffles

Hands-on time:
20 minutes

Overall time:
20 minutes

Eggs Royale Chaffles

Chaffles make the perfect bread base for eggs royale (with smoked salmon) and eggs Benedict (with ham). This is a delicious and satisfying meal packed with goodness. It's is easy to make multiple batches of this recipe if you cook for the whole family!

INGREDIENTS

Chaffles & Topping

Ingredients for 2 Basic Savory Chaffles (page 14)

2 large eggs

Dash of vinegar

2–3 slices (57 g/2 oz) smoked salmon

Optional: pinch of paprika, pinch of chili powder, or 1 teaspoon Sriracha sauce

Hollandaise

2 tablespoons (30 ml) butter, ghee, duck fat, or extra-virgin olive oil

1 large egg yolk

1 teaspoon fresh lemon juice, or more to taste

¼ teaspoon Dijon mustard

Pinch of salt, or more to taste

INSTRUCTIONS

Prepare a batch of the Basic Savory Chaffles by following the instructions on page 14. Let the chaffles cool down.

To make the hollandaise sauce, gently melt the butter and set aside; it should be warm, but not too hot. Fill a medium saucepan with a cup of water and bring to a boil. In a separate bowl, mix the egg yolks with the lemon juice, a dash of water if too thick, Dijon mustard, and salt. Place the bowl over the saucepan filled with water. The water should not touch the bottom of the bowl. Keep mixing until the sauce starts to thicken. Slowly pour the melted butter into the mixture until thick and creamy and stir constantly. If the sauce is too thick, add a splash of water. Set aside and keep warm while you cook the eggs.

Nutrition facts (1 chaffle + topping)

Total carbs:	Fiber:	Net carbs:	Protein:	Fat:	Calories:	Calories from
4.6 g	**1.2 g**	**3.4 g**	**25.3 g**	**38.8 g**	**466 kcal**	**carbs (3%)** **protein (22%)** **fat (75%)**

To poach the eggs, fill a medium saucepan with water and a dash of vinegar. Bring to a boil over high heat. Crack each egg individually into a ramekin or a cup. Using a spoon, create a gentle whirlpool in the water; this will help the egg white wrap around the egg yolk. Slowly lower the egg into the water in the center of the whirlpool. Turn off the heat and cook for 3 to 4 minutes. Use a slotted spoon to remove the egg from the water and place it on a plate. Repeat for all remaining eggs. Once cool, place all the eggs in a sealed container filled with cold water and keep refrigerated for up to 5 days. To reheat the eggs, place them in a mug filled with hot tap water for a couple of minutes. This will be enough to warm them up without overcooking.

Assemble one chaffle (light dish) or two chaffles with smoked salmon, poached egg and a drizzle with hollandaise (about 2 tablespoons/30 ml) per serving). Serve immediately with a pinch of paprika or chili powder or a drizzle of Sriracha (if using).

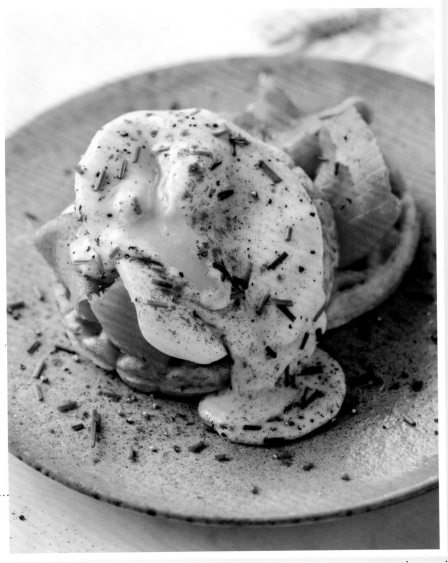

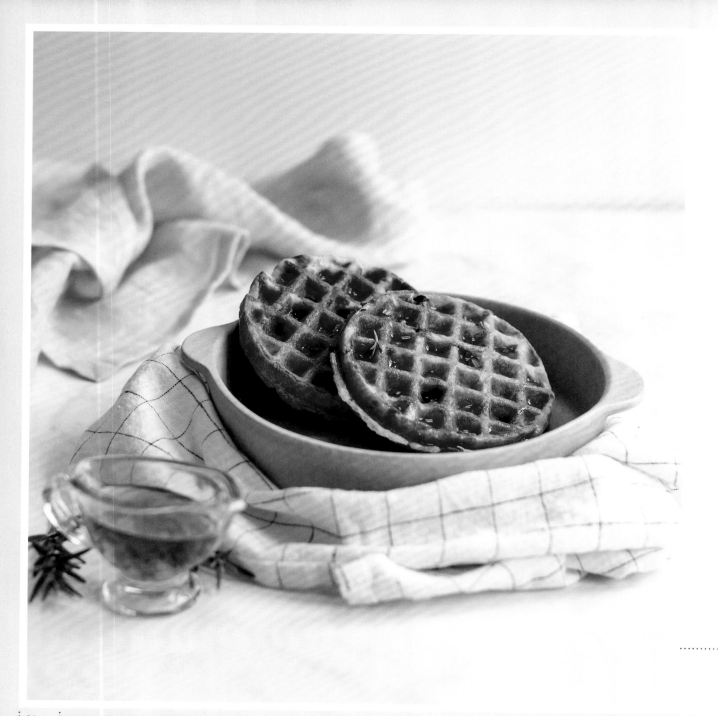

Servings:
2 mini chaffles

Hands-on time:
10 minutes

Overall time:
15 minutes

Rosemary Olive Focaccia Chaffles

This easy focaccia chaffle tastes like the classic Italian bread. It's so rich and wonderful with the addition of fresh rosemary, garlic, and olive oil. Any olives will be delicious, but if you can, use Kalamata olives.

INGREDIENTS

Chaffles
1 large egg white

½ cup (57 g/2 oz) grated mozzarella or other hard cheese

1 teaspoon extra-virgin olive oil

2 tablespoons (12 g/0.4 oz) almond flour

2 tablespoons (10 g/0.4 oz) grated Parmesan

¼ teaspoon gluten-free baking powder

Pinch of black pepper

¼ teaspoon dried rosemary or ½ teaspoon fresh chopped rosemary

6 small pitted (18 g/0.6 oz) black, green, or Kalamata olives, sliced

Topping
1 tablespoon (15 ml) extra-virgin olive oil

¼ teaspoon minced garlic (about ¼ garlic clove)

INSTRUCTIONS

Preheat the waffle maker. Place the egg white, mozzarella, and 1 teaspoon of olive oil in a blender and pulse until smooth (or simply stir to combine). Add the almond flour, Parmesan, baking powder, and black pepper. Blend again. Add the rosemary and olives and stir them through.

To cook the batter, follow the instructions for the Basic Savory Chaffles on page 14. When filling the waffle maker, use half (about 68 g/2.4 oz) of the batter for each chaffle. Although this batter is thick so it's less likely to leak, keep an eye on it (see leakproof tips on page 8).

To make the topping, mix the remaining 1 tablespoon (15 ml) olive oil and minced garlic and let it infuse while the chaffles are cooking.

Let the chaffles cool down slightly. Drizzle the garlic-infused oil on top of the chaffles and serve. They can be stored just like Basic Chaffles (page 8).

Nutrition facts (1 chaffle)

Total carbs:	Fiber:	Net carbs:	Protein:	Fat:	Calories:	Calories from
3.7 g	**1 g**	**2.7 g**	**11.8 g**	**21.4 g**	**251 kcal**	**carbs (4%) protein (19%) fat (77%)**

Mexican Chaffles

These Mexican chaffles are perfect as a quick dinner or breakfast option. Flavored with warming spices and topped with mashed avocado, sour cream, cilantro, and jalapeños, this is the perfect option for busy weeknights.

INGREDIENTS

Chaffles
Ingredients for 2 Basic Savory Chaffles (page 14)

1 tablespoon (15 g/0.5 oz) tomato paste

¼ teaspoon ground cumin

⅛ teaspoon chili powder

¼ teaspoon garlic powder

½ tablespoon chopped fresh cilantro

Topping
½ large (100 g/3.5 oz) avocado, peeled and pitted

Salt and pepper, to taste

3 tablespoons (36 g/1.3 oz) sour cream

½ jalapeño pepper (7 g/ 0.3 oz), sliced and seeds removed, or few slices of pickled jalapeños

2 tablespoons (14 g/0.5 oz) shredded cheese such as cheddar

Optional: chili powder, fresh cilantro, and lime wedges

INSTRUCTIONS

Follow the instructions for the Basic Savory Chaffles on page 14, but also stir in the tomato paste, cumin, chili powder, and garlic powder. If you're using the blending method, place all of the chaffle ingredients in a blender and process until smooth. Then add the chopped cilantro. Otherwise you can simply mix all of the ingredients using a fork.

To make the topping, mash the avocado flesh using a fork. Season with salt and pepper.

Assemble one chaffle (light dish) or two chaffles topped with the mashed avocado, sour cream, jalapeño slices, and cheese. Optionally, sprinkle with chili powder and some cilantro, and serve with lime wedges. Chaffles with no topping can be stored just like Basic Chaffles (page 8).

Nutrition facts (1 chaffle + topping)

Total carbs:	Fiber:	Net carbs:	Protein:	Fat:	Calories:	Calories from
10.3 g	**5 g**	**5.3 g**	**15.6 g**	**31.6 g**	**375 kcal**	**carbs (6%)** **protein (17%)** **fat (77%)**

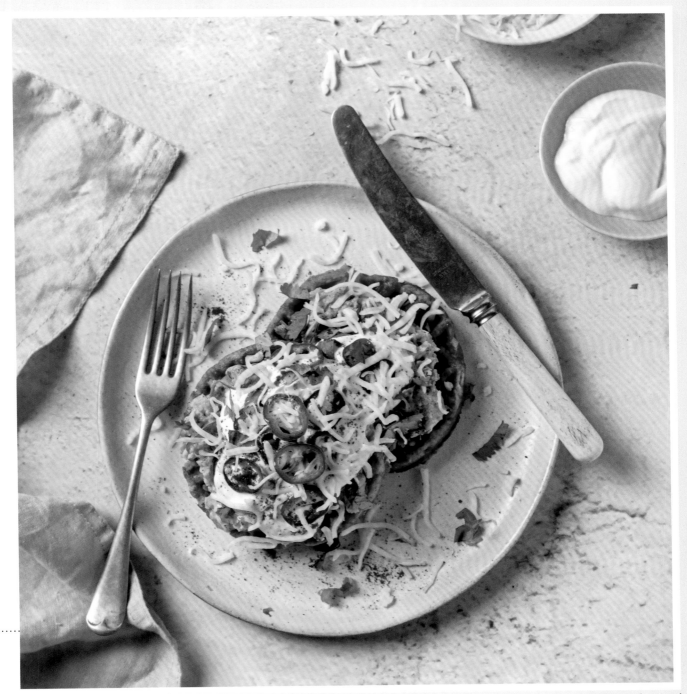

Servings:
2 mini chaffles

Hands-on time:
10 minutes

Overall time:
15 minutes

Quatro Formaggi Pizza Chaffles

This four-cheese chaffle is the ultimate treat for pizza lovers! It's totally up to you which cheese you use, so feel free to try other options such as goat cheese, feta, or Brie.

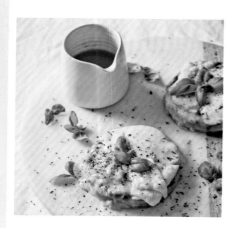

INGREDIENTS

Chaffles
Ingredients for 2 Basic Savory Chaffles, using shredded mozzarella (page 14)

¼ teaspoon dried Italian herbs

Topping
2 tablespoons (30 ml) Marinara Sauce (page 10)

3 tablespoons (15 g/0.5 oz) Parmesan cheese

¼ cup (40 g/1.4 oz) crumbled Gorgonzola cheese

4 slices (60 g/2.1 oz) fresh mozzarella

Fresh basil and black pepper

Optional: 2 teaspoons (10 ml) extra-virgin olive oil

INSTRUCTIONS

Follow the instructions for the Basic Savory Chaffles on page 14, but also add the Italian herbs into the batter before mixing or blending.

Top each chaffle with marinara sauce (preferably the chunky, thicker bits), followed by Parmesan, Gorgonzola, and mozzarella. Place under a broiler and broil for 2 to 3 minutes, or until the cheese has melted. Garnish with fresh basil and black pepper. Optionally, drizzle with olive oil. Serve immediately while still warm. These chaffles can be stored in a sealed container the fridge for up to 3 days. Reheat before serving.

Nutrition facts (1 chaffle + topping)

Total carbs:	Fiber:	Net carbs:	Protein:	Fat:	Calories:	Calories from
7.1 g	**1.9 g**	**5.2 g**	**27 g**	**29.4 g**	**397 kcal**	**carbs (5%)** **protein (27%)** **fat (68%)**

Servings:
2 mini chaffles

Hands-on time:
10 minutes

Overall time:
15 minutes

Pepperoni Pizza Chaffles

Pepperoni pizza in just 15 minutes? This is by far the fastest way to make chaffles that taste like deep-dish pizza. All of the flavor of your favorite Italian takeout with none of the hassle or carbs!

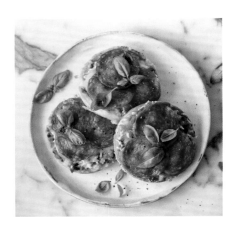

INGREDIENTS

2 Basic Savory Chaffles, ideally made with shredded mozzarella (page 14)

2 tablespoons (30 ml) sugar-free Marinara Sauce (page 10) or tomato paste

¼ cup (28 g/1 oz) grated mozzarella cheese

2 tablespoons (10 g/0.4 oz) grated Parmesan cheese

6 slices (18 g/0.6 oz) pepperoni

Fresh basil

Optional: 2 teaspoons (10 ml) extra-virgin olive oil

INSTRUCTIONS

Follow the instructions for the Basic Savory Chaffles on page 14.

Once cooked, top each waffle with a tablespoon (15 ml) of marinara sauce (preferably the chunky, thicker bits). Add the mozzarella, Parmesan, and pepperoni slices. Place under a broiler for 3 to 5 minutes, until the pepperoni is crisp and the cheese is melted.

Garnish with basil and drizzle with olive oil (if using). These chaffles can be stored in a sealed container in the fridge for up to 3 days. Reheat before serving.

Nutrition facts (1 chaffle + topping)

Total carbs:	Fiber:	Net carbs:	Protein:	Fat:	Calories:	Calories from
6 g	**1.5 g**	**4.5 g**	**19.1 g**	**24.4 g**	**315 kcal**	**carbs (6%) protein (24%) fat (70%)**

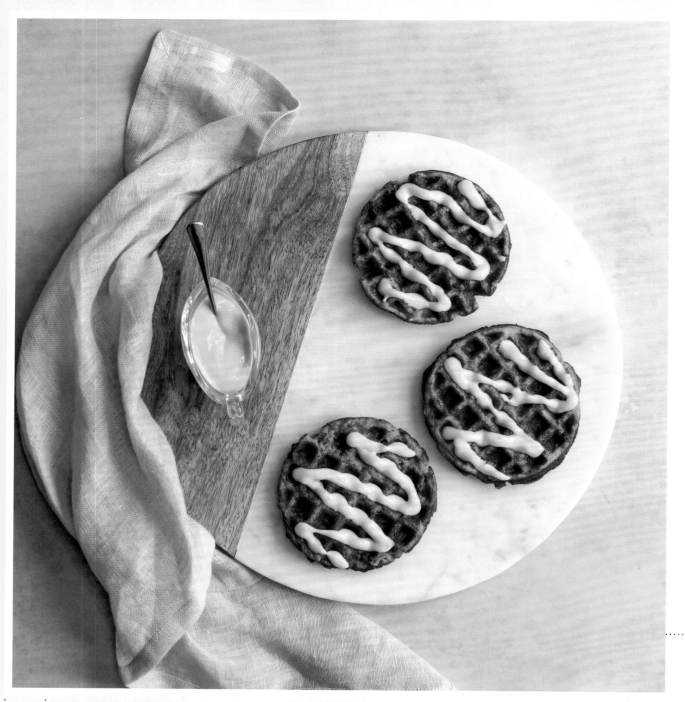

Servings:
3 mini chaffles

Hands-on time:
15 minutes

Overall time:
25 minutes

Meat Lover's Chaffles

This satisfying, cheesy meat chaffle is packed with flavor and protein. It's perfect for lunchboxes and tastes best with guacamole, spicy mayonnaise, or any creamy dip.

INGREDIENTS

3 ounces (85 g) ground beef

1 large egg

½ cup (57 g/2 oz) grated mozzarella or other hard cheese of choice

1 teaspoon Mexican chili paste or tomato paste

¼ teaspoon dried Italian herbs or parsley

¼ cup (23 g/0.8 oz) grated Parmesan cheese

1 teaspoon (3 g/0.2 oz) coconut flour

¼ teaspoon gluten-free baking powder

Optional: A drizzle of Sriracha mayonnaise or plain mayonnaise

INSTRUCTIONS

Place the beef in a hot pan. Cook on medium-high for about 5 minutes, or until opaque and cooked through. Set aside to cool down.

Place all remaining ingredients in a blender or simply mix with a fork. Add the cooked beef and stir through.

To cook the batter, follow the instructions for Basic Savory Chaffles on page 14, but make 3 waffles instead of two. You'll need about one-third (67 g/2.4 oz) of the batter for each chaffle. Although this batter is thick and less likely to leak, keep an eye on it (see leakproof tips on page 8).

Let the chaffles cool down and serve. They can be stored just like Basic Chaffles (page 8).

TIP

✱ You can make your own mayonnaise (using healthy fats such as avocado oil, olive oil, or walnut oil) and Sriracha sauce. There are plenty of recipes at ketodietapp.com/blog!

Nutrition facts (1 chaffle)

Total carbs:	Fiber:	Net carbs:	Protein:	Fat:	Calories:	Calories from
3.1 g	**0.4 g**	**2.6 g**	**21.5 g**	**20 g**	**282 kcal**	**carbs (4%) protein (31%) fat (65%)**

Garlic Bread Chaffles

Waffles and garlic bread—two delicious recipes fused into one! This crispy, fragrant garlic bread chaffle is just like your favorite Italian side.

INGREDIENTS

Chaffles

1 large egg white

¼ cup (28 g/1 oz) grated mozzarella

¼ cup (23 g/0.8 oz) grated Parmesan cheese

2 tablespoons (12 g/0.4 oz) almond flour

1 tablespoon (7 g/0.3 oz) flax meal

¼ teaspoon dried Italian herbs

¼ teaspoon gluten-free baking powder

Topping

2 tablespoons (10 g/0.4 oz) grated Parmesan cheese

1 tablespoon (14 g/0.5 oz) garlic and herb compound butter (see tip)

INSTRUCTIONS

Preheat the waffle maker. You can make these chaffles by blending or mixing. Start with the egg white, mozzarella, and Parmesan. Blend until smooth, add the dry ingredients, and blend again.

To cook the batter, follow the instructions for the Basic Savory Chaffles on page 14. Before adding the batter to the waffle maker, sprinkle the waffle maker with about ½ tablespoon (3 g) of Parmesan cheese per waffle. Spoon half of the batter (about 52 g/1.8 oz) for each chaffle and top with ½ tablespoon of Parmesan. Close the lid and cook until crisp.

Remove from the waffle maker and spread a small amount of the compound butter on each side. Return to the waffle maker and cook for 1 minute. Repeat for the second chaffle. Cut each chaffle into 4 pieces. Serve warm or cold as a side to salads and soups. These chaffles can be stored just like Basic Chaffles (page 8).

Nutrition facts (1 chaffle)

Total carbs:	Fiber:	Net carbs:	Protein:	Fat:	Calories:	Calories from
3.9 g	**1.6 g**	**2.3 g**	**13 g**	**16.9 g**	**217 kcal**	**carbs (4%)** **protein (24%)** **fat (72%)**

TIP

* Homemade compound butter: Place 4 ounces (113 g) of room-temperature butter a medium-sized bowl. Mix the softened butter with 2 tablespoons (30 ml) extra-virgin olive oil, 4 crushed cloves of garlic, and 2 tablespoons (8 g/0.3 oz) chopped parsley or 2 teaspoons dried parsley. Spoon the butter onto a piece of parchment paper. Wrap the butter tightly and roll it to create a log shape. Twist the ends of the paper in opposite directions to seal. Store the butter in the fridge for up to 1 week or freeze for up to 6 months. To freeze it, it helps if you slice it into as many servings as needed. Instead of butter, you can also use ghee, lard, or duck fat. If you use butter alternatives, pour the mixture into a silicone ice cube tray and refrigerate; it's perfect for portion control!

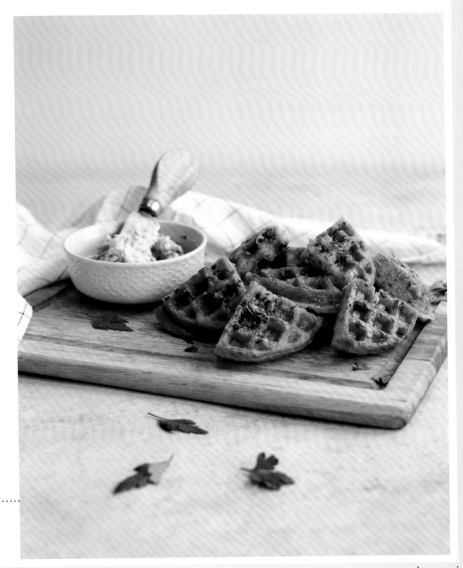

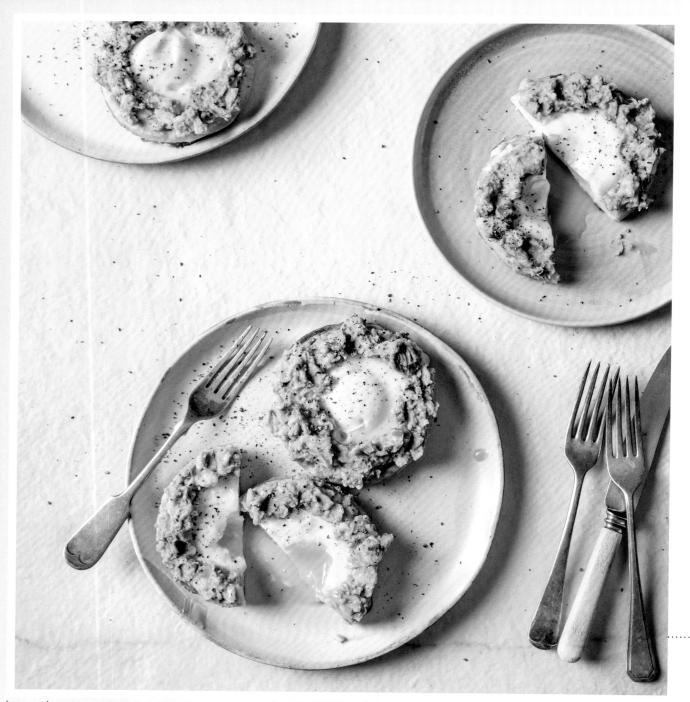

Sweet and Savory Keto Chaffles

Servings:
2 mini chaffles

Hands-on time:
15 minutes

Overall time:
20 minutes

Eggs in a Hole

Who'd have thought you could use chaffles to make eggs in a hole? You can! This chaffle is fun to make, and it's a tasty breakfast meal packed with healthy fats and electrolytes.

INGREDIENTS

Chaffles
Ingredients for 2 Basic Savory Chaffles (page 14)

2 teaspoons (10 ml) ghee or duck fat for greasing

2 large eggs

Topping
1 medium (150 g/5.3 oz) avocado, peeled and pitted

2 tablespoons (30 ml) fresh lime or lemon juice

1 teaspoon extra-virgin olive oil

Salt and pepper, to taste

Optional: 1 tablespoon chopped fresh herbs such as chives, parsley, or spring onion

INSTRUCTIONS

Follow the instructions for the Basic Savory Chaffles on page 14. Once cool, use a 2-inch (5-cm) cookie cutter to create a hole inside each chaffle. (Don't waste these cut-outs. Serve them with the finished meal.)

Place both chaffles in a hot pan greased with ghee. Crack the eggs inside the holes. Fry over medium heat for about 3 minutes, or until the whites are set and the yolks still runny. Optionally, you can add a lid to help them set faster.

Meanwhile, place the avocado in a bowl. Using a fork, mash with the lime juice and olive oil. Season with salt and pepper to taste.

To assemble, place the avocado topping on the chaffle, leaving the runny egg yolk in the center exposed (or simply serve on the side). Eat immediately with a sprinkle of fresh herbs (if using).

Nutrition facts (1 chaffle + topping)

Total carbs:	Fiber:	Net carbs:	Protein:	Fat:	Calories:	Calories from
11.3 g	**6.3 g**	**5 g**	**20.1 g**	**41.4 g**	**484 kcal**	**carbs (4%) protein (17%) fat (79%)**

Cauli Pizza Chaffles

These chaffles taste like the crispiest cauliflower pizza you'll ever have. Pan-roasting the cauli-rice enhances the flavor and also removes any excess moisture so that the cauli-crust can be cooked to perfection with a flavor boost.

INGREDIENTS

4.5 ounces (128 g) cauliflower florets

1 tablespoon (15 ml) ghee or extra-virgin olive oil

1 large egg

1 cup (113 g/4 oz) grated mozzarella

3 tablespoons (19 g/0.7 oz) almond flour or 2 teaspoons (6 g/0.2 oz) coconut flour

¼ teaspoon salt

⅛ teaspoon garlic powder

⅛ teaspoon onion powder

⅛ teaspoon dried Italian herbs

Optional: ½ cup (120 ml) Marinara Sauce (page 10)

INSTRUCTIONS

Grate the cauliflower with a hand grater, or place the florets in a food processor with a grating blade or an S blade and pulse until it looks like rice. Don't overdo it. It only takes a few more seconds to make purée out of your cauliflower. Place the cauliflower on a pan greased with ghee and cook over medium heat for 3 to 5 minutes while stirring. Set aside to cool down.

Place the egg, mozzarella, almond flour, salt, garlic powder, onion powder, and Italian herbs in a bowl. Mix until well combined. Optionally, you can blend these ingredients, but it's not required (page 7). Add the cooked cauli-rice and stir through.

To cook the batter, follow the instructions for the Basic Savory Chaffles on page 14, but make a total of 4 chaffles (about 60 g/ 2.1 oz of raw dough per chaffle). Once cooked and crisp, let the chaffles briefly cool down and serve with Marinara Sauce (if using). These chaffles can be stored just like Basic Chaffles (page 8).

Nutrition facts (1 chaffle)

Total carbs:	Fiber:	Net carbs:	Protein:	Fat:	Calories:	Calories from
4.3 g	**1.2 g**	**3.1 g**	**9.9 g**	**13.1 g**	**172 kcal**	**carbs (7%)** **protein (23%)** **fat (70%)**

TIPS

✳ Add any toppings, such as pepperoni, fresh mozzarella, cooked spinach, mushrooms, or bacon, and broil for 2 to 3 minutes just like Pepperoni Pizza Chaffles (page 31).

✳ Instead of Marinara Sauce, brush with some pesto (page 11) or top with soft goat cheese.

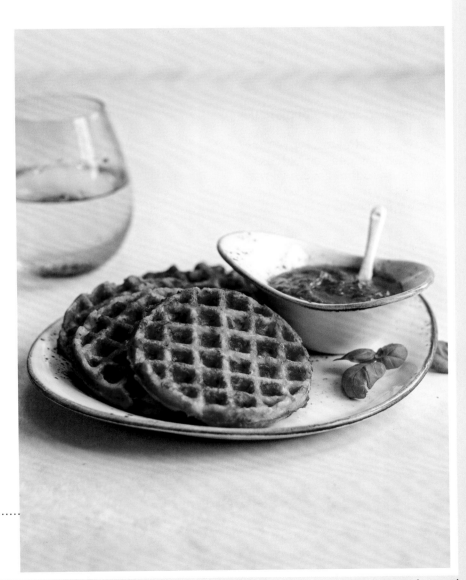

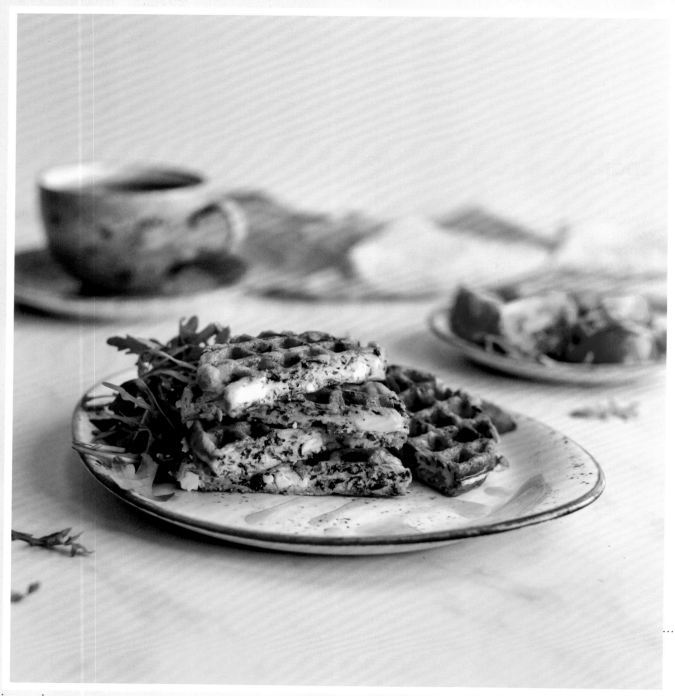

Servings:
3 mini chaffles

Hands-on time:
10 minutes

Overall time:
15 minutes

Spanakopita Chaffles

My cookbook wouldn't be complete without a Greek-inspired dish. These chaffles evoke a popular Greek recipe traditionally made with phyllo dough and filled with spinach and feta. They can be served as an appetizer, a side, or even for breakfast.

INGREDIENTS

1 large egg

½ cup (57 g/2 oz) grated mozzarella

3 tablespoons (15 g/0.5 oz) grated Parmesan cheese

¼ cup (25 g/0.8 oz) almond flour

3 ounces (85 g) frozen spinach, thawed and excess juices squeezed out (about 32 g/ 1.1 oz net weight)

¼ cup (38 g/1.3 oz) crumbled feta cheese

Optional: 1 tablespoon chopped fresh herbs of choice (basil, chives, thyme, and parsley work best)

INSTRUCTIONS

In a bowl, mix the egg, mozzarella, Parmesan cheese, and almond flour until well combined. Optionally, you can blend these ingredients, but it's not required (page 7). Chop the drained spinach and add to the batter. Add the feta and stir through.

To cook the batter, follow the instructions for the Basic Savory Chaffles on page 14, but make a total of 3 chaffles (about 72 g/2.5 oz of raw dough per chaffle). The batter will be very thick and unlikely to overflow, but do keep an eye on it. Cook and crisp up the chaffles; this may take a little longer compared to the Basic Chaffles. Let the chaffles briefly cool down and serve with herbs (if using). These chaffles can be stored just like Basic Chaffles (page 8).

Nutrition facts (1 chaffle)

Total carbs:	Fiber:	Net carbs:	Protein:	Fat:	Calories:	Calories from
4.6 g	**1.7 g**	**2.9 g**	**12.9 g**	**13.8 g**	**189 kcal**	**carbs (6%)** **protein (28%)** **fat (66%)**

Halloumi Chaffle Sticks with Zucchini Hummus

Haloumi and hummus are a match made in heaven! While Halloumi adds a great flavor to the chaffle dipping sticks, roasted zucchini makes a fantastic keto alternative to the traditional hummus made with chickpeas.

INGREDIENTS

Hummus
2 medium (400 g/14.1 oz) zucchini

¼ cup (60 ml) extra-virgin olive oil, divided

Salt and pepper, to taste

¼ cup (63 g/2.2 oz) tahini sesame paste

2 cloves garlic, sliced

3 tablespoons (45 ml) fresh lemon juice

½ teaspoon ground cumin

Hummus Topping
2 tablespoons (30 ml) extra-virgin olive oil

Smoked paprika and/or cumin to sprinkle on top

2 teaspoons (6 g/0.2 oz) white and/or black sesame seeds

Fresh parsley leaves

Halloumi Chaffles
2 large egg whites

1½ cups (170 g/6 oz) grated Halloumi

½ cup (50 g/1.8 oz) almond flour

½ teaspoon gluten-free baking powder

¼ teaspoon ground cumin

Nutrition facts (1 chaffle/3 sticks + about ⅓ cup/80 ml hummus)

Total carbs:	Fiber:	Net carbs:	Protein:	Fat:	Calories:	Calories from
7.7 g	**2.7 g**	**5 g**	**11.6 g**	**31.9 g**	**351 kcal**	**carbs (6%)** **protein (13%)** **fat (81%)**

INSTRUCTIONS

Preheat the oven to 320°F (160°C) fan assisted or 355°F (180°C, or gas mark 4) conventional. Cut the ends of the zucchini, and cut in half lengthwise and down the middle. Arrange on a baking tray cut-side up, brush with 2 tablespoons (30 ml) of olive oil, and sprinkle with salt and pepper. Bake for 30 minutes, or until browned on top.

Once the zucchini is baked, add it to a food processor together with the remaining olive oil, tahini, garlic, lemon juice, and cumin. Blend until smooth. Add the water a tablespoon at a time, up to 3 tablespoons (45 ml) water, at the end if needed for a smoother consistency. Spoon into a flat bowl and use the back of a spoon to create a swirl in the hummus. Drizzle with oil, and sprinkle with spices and seeds.

Using the ingredients for Halloumi chaffles, follow the instructions for the Basic Savory Chaffles on page 14 and make a total of 6 chaffles. To make each chaffle, you'll need about 54 grams/ 1.9 ounces of the batter.

Once cooked and crisp, let the chaffles briefly cool down before slicing each into 3 sticks. Serve with the roasted zucchini hummus. Halloumi chaffles should ideally be served warm. The chaffles can be stored just like Basic Chaffles (page 8). The hummus can be stored in a sealed container in the fridge for up to 5 days.

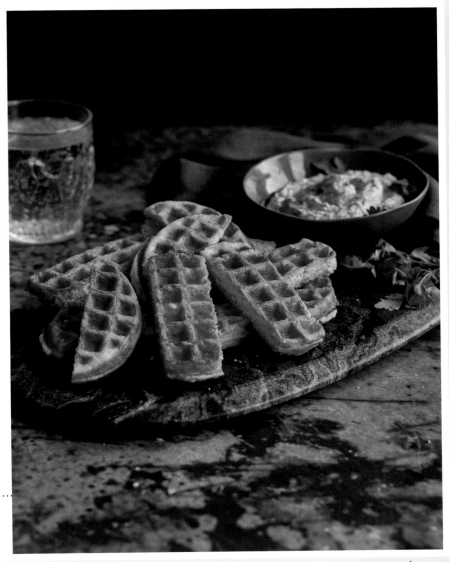

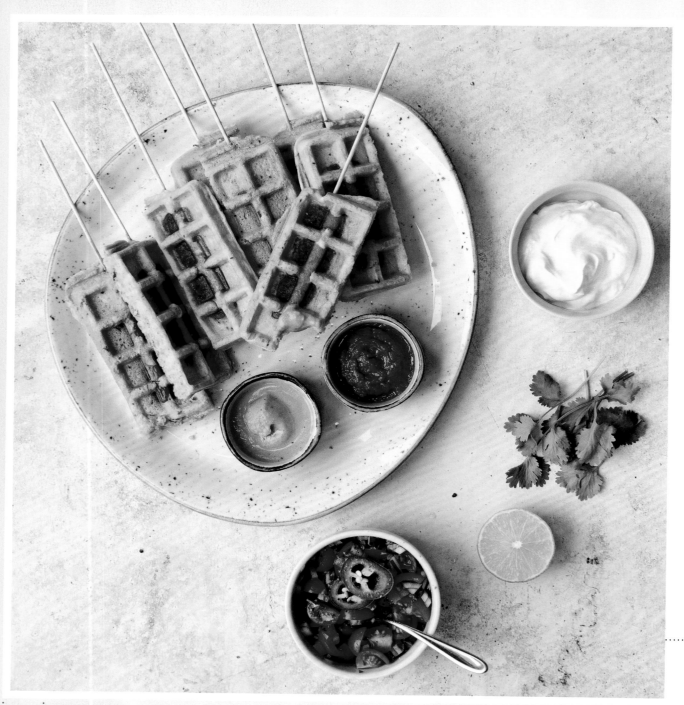

Servings:
8 chaffle corn dogs

Hands-on time:
15 minutes

Overall time:
20 minutes

Chaffle Corn Dogs

A healthier take on a classic American dish. There's no corn and no frying needed when you make a keto version of your favorite snack in a waffle maker!

INGREDIENTS

Chaffles
2 large eggs

1 cup (113 g/4 oz) grated cheddar, mozzarella, or hard cheese of choice (see page 7 for tips)

½ cup (50 g/1.8 oz) almond flour

½ teaspoon gluten-free baking powder

¼ teaspoon garlic powder

¼ teaspoon chili powder

¼ teaspoon red pepper flakes

Filling & Topping
2 hot dogs (142 g/5 oz), quartered, or use cooked gluten-free Italian sausages

Optional: mustard and/or sugar-free ketchup

Optional: sour cream, salsa, jalapeños, shredded cheese, and fresh cilantro

INSTRUCTIONS

Preheat a square Belgian waffle maker (a size that makes 5-inch/12.5-cm waffles). Follow the instructions for the Basic Savory Chaffles on page 14. Preferably, blend all of the ingredients for the batter.

Spoon a very thin layer of the batter (about 34 g/1.2 oz per square) onto the bottom of the hot waffle iron and spread with a spatula or a spoon. Add 2 pieces of hot dog on a stick (like a lollipop) cut-side down on each waffle square. Top each with a bit more batter (about 34 g/1.2 oz per square). Cook until crisp, about 3 to 4 minutes. Transfer to a wire rack and let cool slightly. Continue to make 2 more—each one with 2 hot dog quarters.

Once cool enough to handle, cut them in half to get 2 corn dogs. Optionally, serve with mustard or ketchup for dipping and top them with sour cream, salsa, jalapeños, cheese, and cilantro. These corn dogs can be eaten warm or cold and stored in the fridge for up to 3 days.

TIP
✱ You can make your own mustard and sugar-free ketchup! There are plenty of recipes at ketodietapp.com/blog.

Nutrition facts (1 chaffle corn dog)

Total carbs:	Fiber:	Net carbs:	Protein:	Fat:	Calories:	Calories from
2.4 g	**0.7 g**	**1.7 g**	**8 g**	**12.7 g**	**154 kcal**	**carbs (4%)** **protein (21%)** **fat (75%)**

Servings:
4 mini chaffles + about ⅔ cup (160 ml) gravy

Hands-on time:
20 minutes

Overall time:
25 minutes

Chaffles with Bacon Sausage Gravy

This recipe is my healthier take on a popular American classic. We are using chaffles to replace the traditional biscuits and serving them with a creamy sausage gravy with crisp bacon pieces. Comfort food at its best!

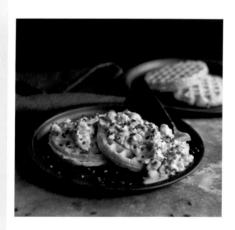

INGREDIENTS

4 Basic Savory Chaffles (page 14)

2 slices (60 g/2.1 oz) bacon, chopped

4 ounces (113 g) gluten-free Italian sausage meat

2 tablespoons (30 g/1.1 oz) full-fat cream cheese

2 tablespoons (30 ml) water or bone broth

1 tablespoon (15 ml) heavy whipping cream

¼ teaspoon onion powder

⅛ teaspoon garlic powder

Salt and pepper, to taste

Optional: Fresh herbs of choice

INSTRUCTIONS

To make the chaffles, follow the instructions for the Basic Savory Chaffles on page 14, but make a total of 4 chaffles. When done, set aside.

Add the bacon pieces and a tablespoon (15 ml) of water to a hot frying pan. Cook over medium-low heat for a few minutes, until the bacon grease is rendered. Then add the sausage meat and cook for about 5 minutes, or until cooked through and crisp.

Add all of the remaining ingredients to make the gravy. Bring to a boil and cook for a few minutes to thicken. Take it off the heat and set aside to cool slightly.

Serve with the chaffles: 1 for a light meal or 2 for a full meal. To store, let the sausage gravy cool down and store in a sealed container for up to 4 days. Reheat before serving.

Nutrition facts (1 chaffle + about 3 tablespoons [45 ml] sausage gravy)

Total carbs:	Fiber:	Net carbs:	Protein:	Fat:	Calories:	Calories from
3.1 g	**0.7 g**	**2.4 g**	**17.6 g**	**31.2 g**	**360 kcal**	**carbs (3%)** **protein (20%)** **fat (77%)**

Caramelized Onion & Brie Chaffles

Looking for a snack packed full of flavor? These chaffles are topped with fragrant, melty cheese on a bed of sweet caramelized onions.

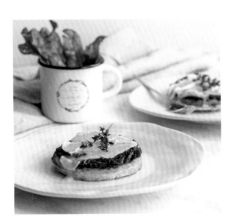

INGREDIENTS

4 Basic Savory Chaffles (page 14)

2 tablespoons (30 ml) ghee, duck fat, or extra-virgin olive oil

2 medium (200 g/7.1 oz) red onions, sliced

2 tablespoons (20 g/0.7 oz) Erythritol, Swerve, or brown sugar substitute

1 tablespoon (15 ml) balsamic vinegar (avoid sweet aged balsamic)

Salt and pepper, to taste

6 ounces (170 g) Brie, sliced

Fresh herbs such as thyme

Optional: crispy bacon slices

INSTRUCTIONS

To make the chaffles, follow the instructions for the Basic Savory Chaffles on page 14, but make a total of 4 chaffles. When done, set aside.

Heat the ghee in a frying pan over medium heat. Add the onions and cook, stirring occasionally, until the onions start to soften, around 12 to 15 minutes. Lower the heat, add the sweetener, vinegar, salt, and pepper, and cook, continuing to stir occasionally, until dark and caramelized.

Top each chaffle with about one-quarter of the caramelized onions. Top with Brie and place under a broiler for 1 to 2 minutes, until the cheese starts to melt. Garnish with fresh herbs and pepper. Serve warm with the optional bacon. To store, let the them cool down and store in a sealed container for up to 3 days. Reheat before serving.

TIP

✱ If you plan to serve these as a more satisfying sandwich, add a few more slices of Brie and top with another chaffle.

Nutrition facts (1 chaffle + topping)

Total carbs:	Fiber:	Net carbs:	Protein:	Fat:	Calories:	Calories from
8.6 g	**1.9 g**	**6.7 g**	**21.7 g**	**37.7 g**	**459 kcal**	**carbs (6%) protein (19%) fat (75%)**

Servings:
6 chaffle kebabs

Hands-on time:
15 minutes

Overall time:
30 minutes

Spiced Veg & Halloumi Chaffle Kebabs

Enjoy the taste of Cyprus in a simple veggie skewer! These tasty chaffle kebabs feature marinated grilled Halloumi and low-carb veggies flavored with warming spices. They are great served with tzatziki, olives, and lemon wedges.

INGREDIENTS

Marinade
2 tablespoons (30 ml) extra-virgin olive oil

1 tablespoon (15 ml) fresh lemon juice

½ teaspoon dried Italian herbs

½ teaspoon paprika

⅛ teaspoon ground cumin

⅛ teaspoon garlic powder

½ teaspoon salt

¼ teaspoon pepper

Kebabs
½ small (140 g/5 oz) zucchini, cut into 1-inch (2.5-cm) pieces

½ small (120 g/4.2 oz) eggplant, cut into 1-inch (2.5-cm) pieces

½ medium (60 g/2.1 oz) red bell pepper, cut into 1-inch (2.5-cm) pieces

8.8 ounces (250 g) Halloumi cheese, cut into 1-inch (2.5-cm) cubes

2 Basic Savory Chaffles (page 14)

INSTRUCTIONS

Preheat the oven to 400°F (200°C) fan assisted or 425°F (220°C, or gas mark 7) conventional. Mix the ingredients to make the marinade. Pour it over the vegetables and Halloumi and toss to cover from all sides. Roast for 15 to 20 minutes, turning halfway through. Optionally, broil for the last 3 minutes to get the Halloumi slightly crisp.

While the vegetables and Halloumi are baking, make the chaffles. Follow the instructions for Basic Savory Chaffles on page 14. Let them cool down slightly and then cut the chaffles into 6 smaller pieces.

When the vegetables and Halloumi are cooked, let them cool slightly before threading them onto the skewers with chaffles in between. If you want to keep this meal simple, serve the grilled vegetables and Halloumi with the chaffles as a side. The grilled vegetables and Halloumi are best eaten fresh, but they can be stored in the fridge for up to 3 days. Reheat before serving.

Nutrition facts (1 kebab)

Total carbs:	Fiber:	Net carbs:	Protein:	Fat:	Calories:	Calories from
4.9 g	**1.6 g**	**3.3 g**	**13.1 g**	**22.1 g**	**265 kcal**	**carbs (5%)** **protein (20%)** **fat (75%)**

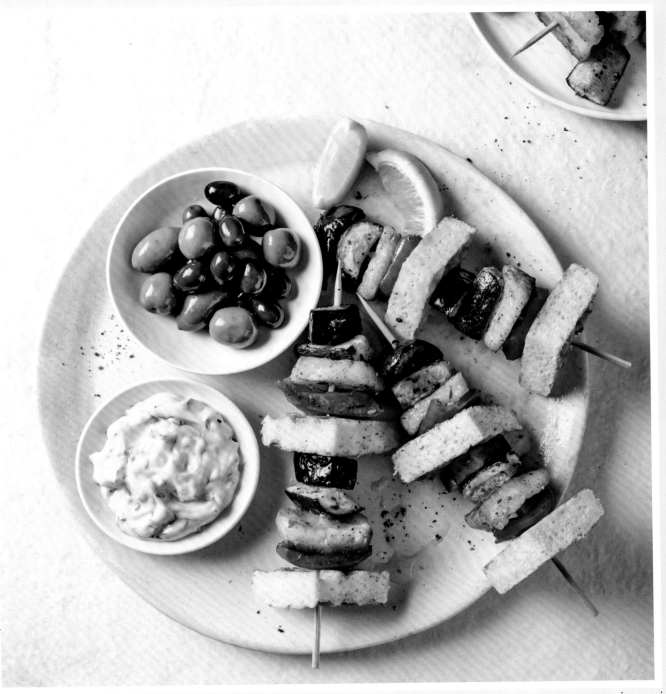

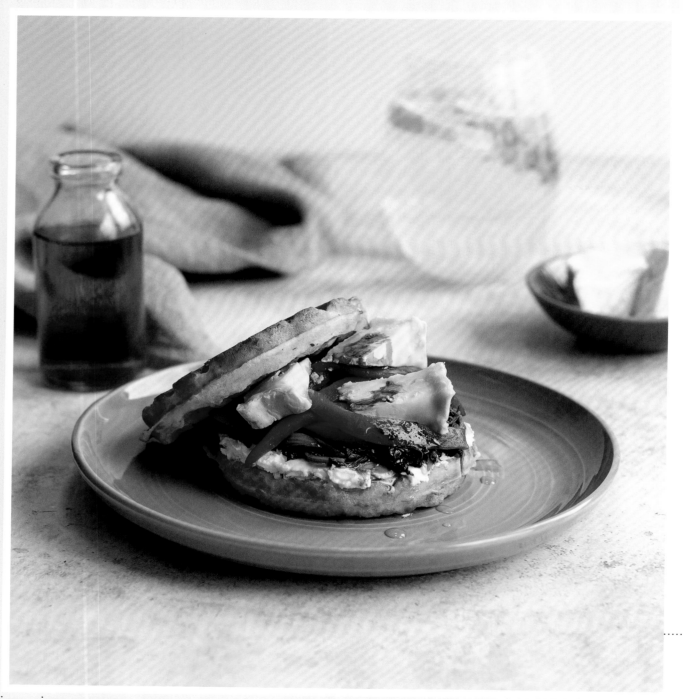

Sweet and Savory Keto Chaffles

Roasted Red Pepper & Goat Cheese Chaffles

These chaffles are inspired by my favorite pizza topping. When I'm too busy to make a regular keto pizza crust, I use chaffles as the base for my toppings and a tasty meal is on the table in a few minutes.

INGREDIENTS

2 Basic Savory Chaffles (page 14)

¼ cup (60 g/2.1 oz) spreadable, soft goat cheese or cream cheese

3 ounces (85 g) frozen spinach, thawed and excess juices squeezed out (about 33 g/ 1.2 oz net weight)

¼ cup (45 g/1.6 oz) roasted red pepper, sliced

6 slices (60 g/2.1 oz) semi-soft goat cheese, sliced

½ teaspoon balsamic vinegar (avoid sweet aged balsamic)

2 teaspoons (10 ml) extra-virgin olive oil

INSTRUCTIONS

Follow the instructions for the Basic Savory Chaffles on page 14. When done, set aside.

Spread the soft goat cheese on the chaffles. Top each with drained spinach, roasted red pepper, and goat cheese. Drizzle with drops of balsamic vinegar and olive oil. Serve immediately or store in the fridge for up to 1 day.

TIP

* You can serve this as a sandwich. To do that, simply put all of the topping on one chaffle and top with the second chaffle.

Nutrition facts (1 chaffle + topping)

Total carbs:	Fiber:	Net carbs:	Protein:	Fat:	Calories:	Calories from
6.4 g	**2.7 g**	**3.7 g**	**26 g**	**38.4 g**	**470 kcal**	**carbs (3%) protein (22%) fat (75%)**

Full English Breakfast Chaffles

The traditional English-style breakfast is the kind of dish I can have pretty much every single day without getting bored. What's not to love about a warm chaffle topped with melty cheese, crispy bacon, creamy poached egg, and roasted sweet cherry tomatoes? All without the carb-heavy ingredients such as beans, black pudding, fried potatoes, and bread.

INGREDIENTS

1 Basic Savory Chaffle (page 14)

2 thin-cut slices (30 g/1.1 oz) bacon

4 roasted cherry tomatoes (20 g/0.7 oz) on the vine

1 slice (28 g/1 oz) of cheddar cheese or hard cheese of choice

1 large egg, poached or fried (see page 25 for instructions)

Salt and black pepper, to taste

1 teaspoon extra-virgin olive oil

Optional: sliced avocado, roasted mushrooms, or cooked spinach

INSTRUCTIONS

Follow the instructions for the Basic Savory Chaffles on page 14. You will only need 1 chaffle.

Start by crisping up the bacon pieces. To do that, put the bacon in a hot pan and add 1 or 2 tablespoons (15 or 30 ml) of water. Cook for over medium-low heat for a few minutes until the bacon grease is rendered. Push the bacon to the side and add the cherry tomatoes. Fry for 2 to 3 minutes over high heat, until blisters appear. Transfer to a plate.

Place a chaffle into the pan in which you cooked the bacon and add a slice of cheese on top. Cook until the cheese starts to melt and then transfer to a plate.

To assemble, top with bacon slices, poached egg, and roasted tomatoes, and season with salt and black pepper. Drizzle with olive oil and serve warm with avocado, mushrooms, or spinach (if using).

Nutrition facts (1 chaffle + topping)

Total carbs:	Fiber:	Net carbs:	Protein:	Fat:	Calories:	Calories from
5.4 g	**1.4 g**	**4 g**	**29.2 g**	**44.5 g**	**537 kcal**	**carbs (3%)** **protein (22%)** **fat (75%)**

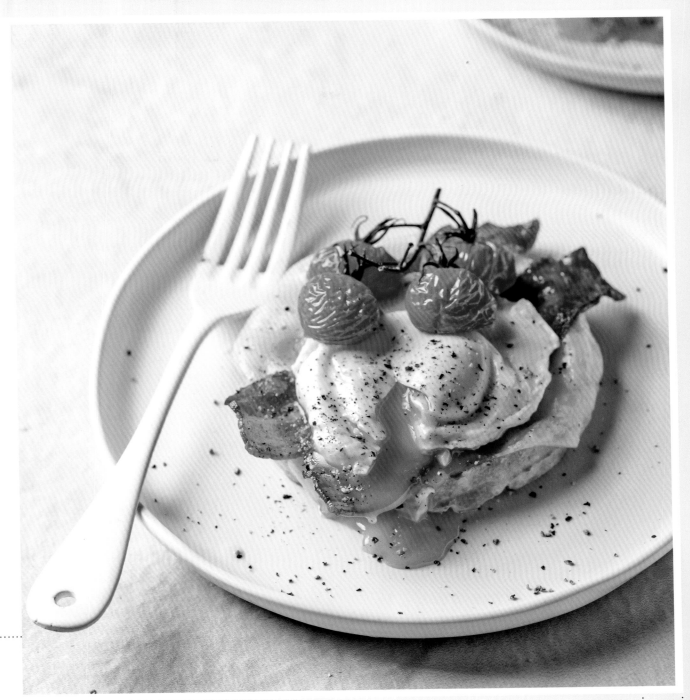

Avocado & Sausage Chaffle Stacks

Healthy eating doesn't have to be lacking creativity. These chaffle stacks look cute, are super nutritious, and are packed flavor.

INGREDIENTS

Chaffles
Ingredients for 2 Basic Savory Chaffles (page 14)

½ teaspoon paprika

Avocado Smash
½ large (100 g/3.5 oz) avocado

Salt and pepper, to taste

Topping
2 teaspoons (9 g) ghee or duck fat, divided

6 ounces (170 g) gluten-free Italian sausage meat

2 large eggs

Black pepper

Optional: A drizzle of Sriracha mayonnaise or plain mayonnaise

INSTRUCTIONS

Follow the instructions for the Basic Savory Chaffles on page 14, but also include paprika when mixing or blending the batter. When the chaffles are done, set aside to cool down.

To prepare the avocado smash, halve the avocado and scoop it into a bowl. Add the salt and pepper. Mash with a fork and set aside.

Heat a pan greased with half of the ghee over medium heat. Using your hands, create two small patties from the sausage meat. Place on the pan and cook undisturbed for 2 to 3 minutes. Flip to the other side and cook for 1 to 2 minutes. Set aside.

Grease the same hot pan with the remaining ghee and crack in the eggs. Cook over medium-high heat until the egg whites are cooked through and the egg yolks are still runny.

When done, top each chaffle with a sausage patty, followed by the avocado smash and fried egg. Season with black pepper to taste and top with the mayonnaise (if using). Eat immediately.

Nutrition facts (1 chaffle stack, served with 1 chaffle)

Total carbs:	Fiber:	Net carbs:	Protein:	Fat:	Calories:	Calories from
9.4 g	**5.2 g**	**4.2 g**	**33.8 g**	**50.6 g**	**618 kcal**	**carbs (3%)** **protein (22%)** **fat (75%)**

TIPS

✱ For a more satisfying meal, you can serve this as a sandwich. To do that, you'll need an extra 2 chaffles (one for each stack).

✱ To save time, prepare the avocado smash and fry the sausage patties in advance and keep in a sealed container for up to 3 days. Poached eggs can be stored in the fridge in a bowl filled with water for up to 3 days.

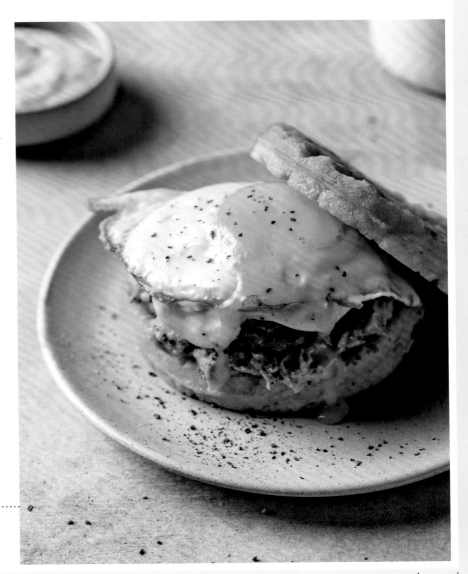

Servings:
2 chaffle stacks

Hands-on time:
15 minutes

Overall time:
20 minutes

Taco Chaffle Stacks

These chaffles are perfect for building lunchboxes. Prepare the individual components in a few minutes and have them ready in the fridge. You've got a quick breakfast, lunch, or dinner sorted!

INGREDIENTS

Ingredients for 2 Basic Savory Chaffles (page 14)

1 teaspoon ghee, duck fat, or lard

6 ounces (170 g) ground beef

2 tablespoons (30 ml) taco sauce or 1 teaspoon sugar-free taco seasoning

2 tablespoons (14 g/0.5 oz) grated cheddar

2 tablespoons (30 ml) sour cream

½ medium (75 g/2.7 oz) avocado, peeled, pitted, and sliced

4 pitted olives (12 g/0.4 oz)

Optional: sliced jalapeños, fresh cilantro, and lime wedges

INSTRUCTIONS

Follow the instructions for the Basic Savory Chaffles on page 14. When the chaffles are done, set aside.

Heat a pan greased with ghee over medium-high heat. Add the beef and cook for 5 to 7 minutes, until opaque and lightly crisped. Add the taco sauce and cook for 1 minute.

To assemble, top each chaffle with half of the ground taco beef and add the cheddar, sour cream, avocado, and olives, plus any optional toppings. Serve warm.

Nutrition facts (1 chaffle + topping)

Total carbs:	Fiber:	Net carbs:	Protein:	Fat:	Calories:	Calories from
8.6 g	**4.3 g**	**4.3 g**	**29.8 g**	**49 g**	**589 kcal**	**carbs (3%)** **protein (21%)** **fat (76%)**

TIP

✱ You can make your own taco sauce (about 1¾ cups/415 ml). Place the following ingredients in a saucepan: 1 cup (240 ml) tomato sauce, 2 tablespoons (30 ml) apple cider vinegar, 1 tablespoon (5 g/0.2 oz) ground cumin, ½ cup (120 ml) water, 1 teaspoon onion powder, ½ teaspoon garlic powder, 1 teaspoon dried oregano, 1 teaspoon Mexican chile powder of choice, 1 teaspoon sweet or smoked paprika, 2 to 3 teaspoons erythritol or Swerve (or 3 to 6 drops of stevia), ¼ teaspoon cayenne pepper, and 1 teaspoon salt or to taste. Bring to a boil and cook over medium-low heat for 7 to 10 minutes, until reduced and thickened slightly. Store in the fridge in a sealed jar for up to 1 week or freeze in an ice cube tray for up to 6 months.

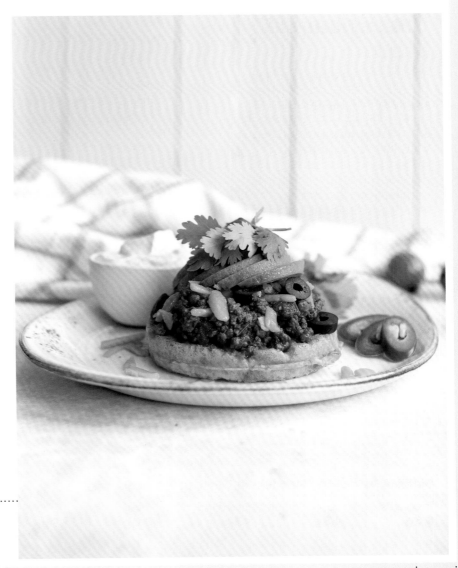

Cheesy Veggie Stacks

I'll be honest. Veggie burgers used to be the last item I would look at on a restaurant's menu. Well, let me introduce you to the most delicious veggie patties! This is how I make meatless burgers that are hearty and flavorful, and unlike most veggie recipes, these are packed with protein.

INGREDIENTS
2 Basic Savory Chaffles (page 14)

Fritters
1 small (150 g/5.3 oz) zucchini

5.3 ounces (150 g) frozen spinach, thawed and squeezed dry (about 57 g/2 oz net weight)

1 large egg

¼ teaspoon salt, or to taste

⅛ teaspoon black pepper, or to taste

1 tablespoon (8 g/0.3 oz) coconut flour

1 teaspoon onion powder

¼ teaspoon garlic powder

⅛ teaspoon red pepper flakes

¼ cup (20 g/0.7 oz) grated Parmesan cheese or 3 tablespoons (25 g/0.9 oz) crumbled feta cheese

2 teaspoons (10 ml) ghee or duck fat for frying

Mint Dressing
1 tablespoon (15 ml) mayonnaise made from healthy fats such as avocado oil

1 teaspoon fresh lemon juice

2 tablespoons (30 ml) full-fat yogurt

1 tablespoon (3 g/0.2 oz) chopped fresh mint or ½ teaspoon dried mint

Salt and pepper, to taste

Optional: 1 cup (10 g/0.4 oz) arugula, spinach, or lettuce

Nutrition facts (1 chaffle stack, served with 1 chaffle)

Total carbs:	Fiber:	Net carbs:	Protein:	Fat:	Calories:	Calories from
13.1 g	**5.4 g**	**7.8 g**	**25.1 g**	**36.7 g**	**472 kcal**	**carbs (7%) protein (22%) fat (71%)**

INSTRUCTIONS

To make the chaffles, follow the instructions for the Basic Savory Chaffles on page 14. When the chaffles are done, set aside.

To make the veggie patties, grate the zucchini and place it in a bowl lined with cheesecloth. Twist the cheesecloth around the zucchini and squeeze out as much liquid out as you can. You should end up with 90–100 grams of drained zucchini.

In a mixing bowl, mix together the zucchini, spinach, egg, salt, and pepper. Add the coconut flour and stir again. Add the onion powder, garlic powder, red pepper flakes, and cheese. Mix through.

Heat a large pan greased with ghee over medium heat. Once hot, shape 2 large burgers with your hands and place them in the hot pan. Cook them for 4 to 5 minutes per side, until golden and crisp.

To make the dressing, place the mayonnaise, lemon juice, yogurt, mint, salt, and pepper in a small bowl. Mix to combine. Season to taste.

To assemble, place greens of your choice on top of two chaffles (optional), and add a veggie patty on top of each chaffle. Drizzle each patty with the dressing and serve warm. The patties and dressing can be stored in a sealed jar in the fridge for up to 3 days. Reheat the patties on a pan or in a microwave before assembling the stacks.

TIP

* For an even more satisfying meal, you can serve this as a sandwich. To do that, you'll need an extra two chaffles (one for each burger).

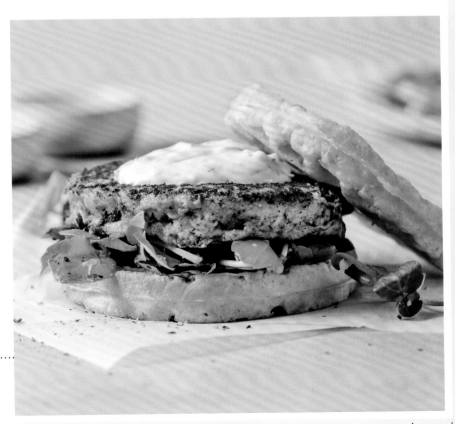

Servings:
2 chaffle stacks

Hands-on time:
15 minutes

Overall time:
25 minutes

Cheeseburger Chaffle Stacks

Did you know you could use chaffles instead of burger buns? Add burger dressing, melty cheese, and pickles and you've got the perfect keto-friendly alternative to your favorite takeout. This meal is a nutritious option for those who practice intermittent fasting.

INGREDIENTS

2 Basic Savory Chaffles (page 14)

Dressing

2 tablespoons (30 g/1.1 oz) mayonnaise made from healthy fats such as avocado oil

1 tablespoon (15 g/1.1 oz) tomato paste

1½ teaspoons fresh lemon juice

Salt and pepper, to taste

2 teaspoons chopped fresh chives or parsley

Burgers

8.8 ounces (250 g) ground beef (about 125 g/4.4 oz per patty)

⅛ teaspoon garlic powder

1 teaspoon onion powder

½ teaspoon apple cider vinegar

½ teaspoon salt

½ teaspoon pepper

2 teaspoons (10 ml) ghee or duck fat for frying

2 slices (40 g/1.4 oz) provolone or cheddar cheese

Topping

4 leaves (40 g/1.4 oz) baby gem lettuce or greens of choice

4 slices (80 g/2.8 oz) medium tomato

4 slices (20 g/0.7 oz) medium red onion

Optional: sugar-free pickles

Nutrition facts (1 chaffle stack, served with 1 chaffle)

Total carbs:	Fiber:	Net carbs:	Protein:	Fat:	Calories:	Calories from
9.3 g	**2.6 g**	**6.7 g**	**40 g**	**61.4 g**	**747 kcal**	**carbs (4%)** **protein (22%)** **fat (74%)**

INSTRUCTIONS

To make the chaffles, follow the instructions for the Basic Savory Chaffles on page 14. When the chaffles are done, set aside.

To make the dressing, place the mayonnaise, tomato paste, lemon juice, salt, pepper, and chives in a small bowl. Mix to combine. Season to taste.

To make the burger patties, combine the beef, garlic powder, onion powder, vinegar, salt, and pepper in a bowl. Divide the ground meat into 2 parts (about 125 g/4.4 oz each). Use your hands to shape each piece into a loose patty, about 3½ inches (9 cm) in diameter and ½ to ¾ inch (1¼ to 2 cm) thick. Pierce the patties with a fork several times. This will loosen the patties and help them cook evenly without curling or getting tough while enabling maximum caramelization.

Heat a large pan greased with the ghee over high heat. Use a spatula to transfer the patties to the hot pan. Cook for 2 to 3 minutes, and then flip over with the spatula and cook for an additional 2 to 3 minutes. Place the cheese on top of the patties for the last minute of the cooking process. Set aside.

To assemble, place the lettuce on two chaffles. Top with tomato, onion, and beef patties, and drizzle with the prepared dressing. Serve warm with pickles (if using).

TIPS

* For an even more satisfying meal, you can serve this as a sandwich. To do that, you'll need an extra two chaffles (one for each burger).

* Dressing variations: Swap the herbs for grated pickle. Swap the tomato paste for Siracha. Add a pinch of smoked chili powder and use lime juice instead of lemon juice.

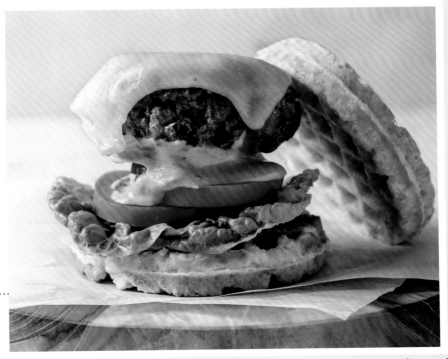

Servings:
2 chaffle burgers

Hands-on time:
15 minutes

Overall time:
25 minutes

Salmon Chaffle Burgers

There are endless ways to make fish cakes, and they can be adjusted to almost any preference. These salmon patties are bigger and seriously moreish. Add lemon dressing and you have an easy, satisfying meal.

INGREDIENTS

4 Basic Savory Chaffles (page 14)

Salmon Patties

8.8 ounces (250 g) canned salmon

1 large egg

¼ cup (25 g/0.9 oz) almond flour or 1 tablespoon (8 g/0.3 oz) coconut flour

1 tablespoon (4 g/0.2 oz) chopped fresh herbs such as dill and/or parsley

1 small (10 g/0.4 oz) spring onion, chopped

1 clove garlic, minced

½ teaspoon paprika

¼ teaspoon salt

Pinch of black pepper

2 teaspoons (10 ml) ghee or duck fat for frying

Lemon Dressing

3 tablespoons (45 ml) mayonnaise made from healthy fats such as avocado oil

1½ teaspoons fresh lemon juice

½ teaspoon fresh lemon zest

1 teaspoon extra-virgin olive oil

¼ teaspoon Dijon mustard

Salt and pepper, to taste

1 teaspoon chopped fresh herbs such as parsley and/or dill

Topping

2–4 lettuce (40 g/1.4 oz), arugula, or spinach leaves

Optional: lemon wedges

Nutrition facts (1 chaffle burger)

Total carbs:	Fiber:	Net carbs:	Protein:	Fat:	Calories:	Calories from
11.8 g	**4.4 g**	**7.4 g**	**64.2 g**	**74.1 g**	**953 kcal**	**carbs (3%)** **protein (27%)** **fat (70%)**

INSTRUCTIONS

To make the chaffles, follow the instructions for the Basic Savory Chaffles on page 14. When the chaffles are done, set aside.

To make the patties, place all the ingredients except the ghee in a mixing bowl and combine. Divide the mixture into 2 parts (about 170 g/6 oz per patty) and use your hands to form large fish cakes.

Heat a large pan greased with the ghee over medium heat. Once hot, add both patties and cook on each side until crisp for 5 to 7 minutes per side. Use a spatula to flip them over. (Do not force the patties out of the pan; if a patty doesn't release when you try to flip it, cook it for a few more seconds until it's crisp and ready to flip.) Set the cooked patties aside.

While the patties are cooking, prepare the dressing by combining the mayonnaise, lemon juice, lemon zest, olive oil, Dijon mustard, salt, pepper, and herbs. Set aside.

To assemble, place the lettuce on both chaffles. Top with tomato, onion, and salmon patties, drizzle with the prepared dressing, and top with the remaining chaffles. Serve warm with lemon wedges (if using).

TIP

✳ This meal is great for those who practice intermittent fasting. If a full serving is too much for you, either serve it as a stack (without the top chaffle) or serve only half of the burger alongside any salad.

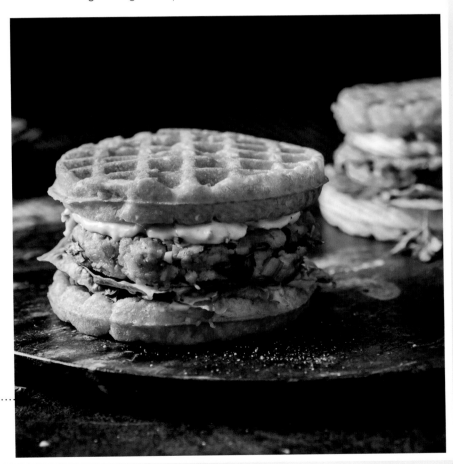

Servings:
2 chaffle burgers

Hands-on time:
15 minutes

Overall time:
25 minutes

Crab Cake Chaffle Burgers

Crab cakes are a great seafood alternative to beef patties in burgers, so why not serve them on top of a cheesy chaffle? Feel free to serve with a side of coleslaw or dressed greens.

INGREDIENTS
4 Basic Savory Chaffles (page 14)

Crab Cakes
6 ounces (170 g) crabmeat

1 large egg

2 tablespoons (30 ml) mayonnaise made from healthy fats such as avocado oil

1 teaspoon Dijon mustard

½ teaspoon Sriracha sauce or chopped chile pepper

1½ tablespoon (11 g/0.4 oz) flax meal or coconut flour

1 small (10 g/0.4 oz) chopped spring onion

1½ teaspoons chopped dill or ½ teaspoon dried dill

¼ teaspoon onion powder

⅛ teaspoon garlic powder

¼ teaspoon salt

Pinch of black pepper

2 teaspoons (10 ml) ghee or duck fat for frying

Tomato Dressing
2 tablespoons (30 ml) mayonnaise made from healthy fats such as avocado oil

2 teaspoons (10 ml) tomato paste

1 teaspoon fresh lemon juice

Optional: ⅛ teaspoon prepared horseradish

Topping
2 to 4 lettuce (40 g/1.4 oz), arugula, or spinach leaves

Optional: more fresh herbs, chilies, and lemon wedges

Nutrition facts (1 chaffle burger)

Total carbs:	Fiber:	Net carbs:	Protein:	Fat:	Calories:	Calories from
11.2 g	**4.7 g**	**6.6 g**	**45.8 g**	**68.1 g**	**821 kcal**	**carbs (3%)** **protein (22%)** **fat (75%)**

INSTRUCTIONS

To make the chaffles, follow the instructions for the Basic Chaffles on page 14. When the chaffles are done, set aside.

To make the patties, place all the ingredients except the ghee in a mixing bowl and combine. Divide the mixture into 2 parts (about 140 g/5 oz per patty) and use your hands to form large fish cakes.

Heat a large pan greased with the ghee over medium heat. Once hot, add both patties and cook until crisp on each side, for about 5 minutes per side. Use a spatula to flip them over. (Do not force the patties out of the pan; if a patty doesn't release when you try to flip it, cook it for a few more seconds until it's crisp and ready to flip.) Set the cooked patties aside.

While the patties are cooking, prepare the dressing by simply combining the mayonnaise, tomato paste, lemon juice, and horseradish. Set aside.

To assemble, place the lettuce on both chaffles, add the patties, drizzle with the prepared dressing, and add any herbs, chilies, or lemon (if using). Top with the remaining chaffle and serve warm.

TIP

✱ To adjust the serving size, check the tip for intermittent fasting on page 63.

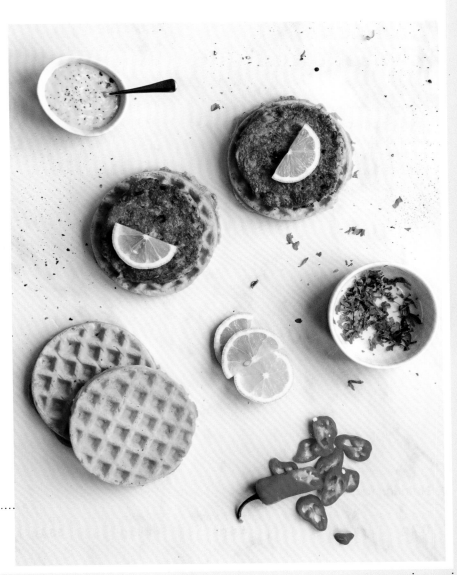

Spicy Fish Chaffle Stacks

If you prefer your fish cakes with a spicy kick like I do, give these a try. You can always adjust the heat by using mild curry powder and paprika instead of chili. Then swap the Sriracha for tomato paste and you've got a kid-friendly meal!

INGREDIENTS

4 Basic Savory Chaffles (page 14)

Fish Cakes

8.8 ounces (250 g) raw cod, haddock, or other white fish, skinless and boneless

1 large egg

2 tablespoons (16 g/0.6 oz) coconut flour

¼ teaspoon salt

Pinch of black pepper

1 teaspoon red pepper flakes, plus more for serving

1 clove garlic, minced

2 teaspoons curry powder (mild or spicy to taste)

½ teaspoon ground cumin

½ teaspoon paprika

1 medium (15 g/0.5 oz) spring onion, chopped

1 tablespoon (4 g/0.2 oz) chopped fresh cilantro or parsley

2 teaspoons (10 ml) ghee or duck fat for frying

Sriracha Mayo

2 tablespoons (30 ml) mayonnaise made from healthy fats such as avocado oil

2 teaspoons (10 ml) Sriracha sauce

Topping

2–4 lettuce leaves (40 g/1.4 oz) or other greens such as spinach

Nutrition facts (1 chaffle stack, served with 1 chaffle)

Total carbs:	Fiber:	Net carbs:	Protein:	Fat:	Calories:	Calories from
11.3 g	**5.3 g**	**6 g**	**40.6 g**	**36.5 g**	**534 kcal**	**carbs (5%)** **protein (32%)** **fat (63%)**

INSTRUCTIONS

To make the chaffles, follow the instructions for the Basic Chaffles on page 14. When the chaffles are done, set aside.

Place all the ingredients except the spring onion, cilantro, and ghee in a blender. Process until smooth. Add the spring onion and cilantro and stir through.

To make the patties, place the fish mixture in a mixing bowl. Divide the mixture into 2 parts (about 175 g/6.2 oz per patty) and use your hands to form large fish cakes.

Heat a large pan greased with the ghee over medium heat. Once hot, add both patties and cook on each side until crisp, for 5 to 7 minutes per side. Use a spatula to flip them over. (Do not force the patties out of the pan; if a patty doesn't release when you try to flip it, cook it for a few more seconds until it's crisp and ready to flip.) Set the cooked patties aside.

While the patties are cooking, prepare the dressing by simply combining the mayonnaise and Sriracha. Set aside.

To assemble, place the lettuce on both chaffles. Top with spicy fish patties and drizzle with the prepared Sriracha mayo. Serve warm.

TIP

✱ For an even more satisfying meal, you can serve this as a sandwich. To do that, you'll need an extra two chaffles (one for each burger).

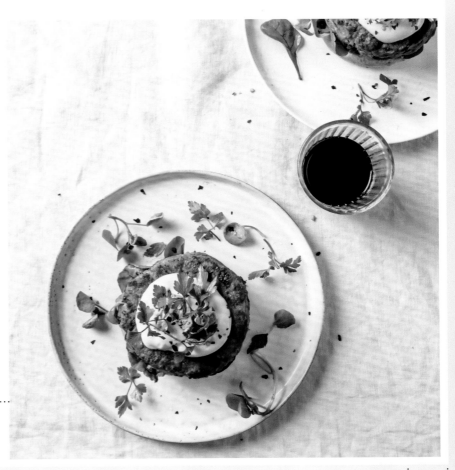

Harissa Lamb Chaffle Stacks

There are flavors that just work together every single time—this meal is a fusion of two of my favorite cuisines. Deliciously juicy Moroccan-style harissa-flavored burgers are drizzled with creamy Greek-style feta-and-herb dip. Serve these with satisfying chaffles and fresh crispy veggies, and you've got a satisfying meal prepped in less than half an hour.

INGREDIENTS

2 Basic Savory Chaffles (page 14)

Lamb Burgers
8.8 ounces (250 g) ground lamb

2 tablespoons (30 ml) harissa paste

¼ teaspoon salt

Pinch of black pepper

2 teaspoons (10 ml) ghee or duck fat for frying

Creamy Feta Dip
⅓ cup (80 ml) sour cream

2 tablespoons (8 g/0.3 oz) chopped fresh herbs such as dill, parsley, and/or mint

2 teaspoons (10 ml) fresh lemon juice

¼ teaspoon ground cumin

¼ cup (38 g/1.3 oz) crumbled feta cheese

Salt and pepper, to taste

Topping
1 cup (10 g/0.4 oz) arugula or other leafy greens of choice

1 small (85 g/3 oz) cucumber, julienned into wide noodles or sliced

4 slices (20 g/0.7 oz) medium red onion

2 slices (40 g/1.4 oz) medium tomato

Nutrition facts (1 chaffle stack, served with 1 chaffle)

Total carbs:	Fiber:	Net carbs:	Protein:	Fat:	Calories:	Calories from
12.3 g	**3.3 g**	**9.1 g**	**38.8 g**	**57.9 g**	**715 kcal**	**carbs (5%)** **protein (22%)** **fat (73%)**

INSTRUCTIONS

To make the chaffles, follow the instructions for the Basic Chaffles on page 14. When the chaffles are done, set aside.

To make the patties, combine the lamb with harissa, salt, and pepper. Divide the ground meat into 2 parts (about 140 g/ 5 oz each). Use your hands to shape each part into a loose burger, about 3½ inches (9 cm) in diameter and ½ to ¾ inch (1¼ to 2 cm) thick. Pierce the patties with a fork several times. This will loosen the patties and help them cook evenly without curling or getting tough while enabling maximum caramelization.

Heat a large pan greased with the ghee over high heat. Use a spatula to transfer the burgers to the hot pan. Cook for 2 to 3 minutes, and then flip over with the spatula and cook for an additional 2 to 3 minutes. Set aside.

While the patties are cooking, prepare the creamy feta dip by simply mixing the sour cream, herbs, lemon juice, cumin, feta, salt, and pepper. Set aside.

To assemble, place the greens, lamb burgers, cucumber, onion, and tomatoes on both chaffles. Serve warm with the prepared dip.

TIPS

* For an even more satisfying meal, you can serve this as a sandwich. To do that, you'll need an extra two chaffles (one for each burger).

* You can make your own harissa paste. There are plenty of recipes at ketodietapp.com/blog!

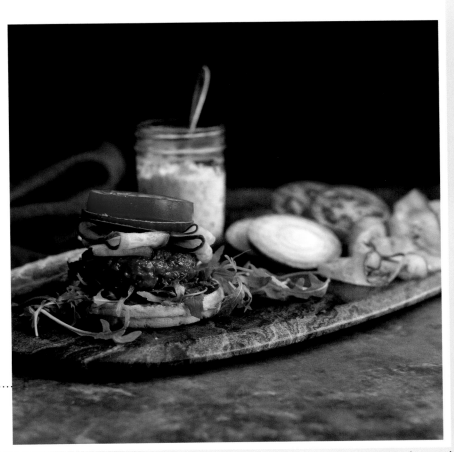

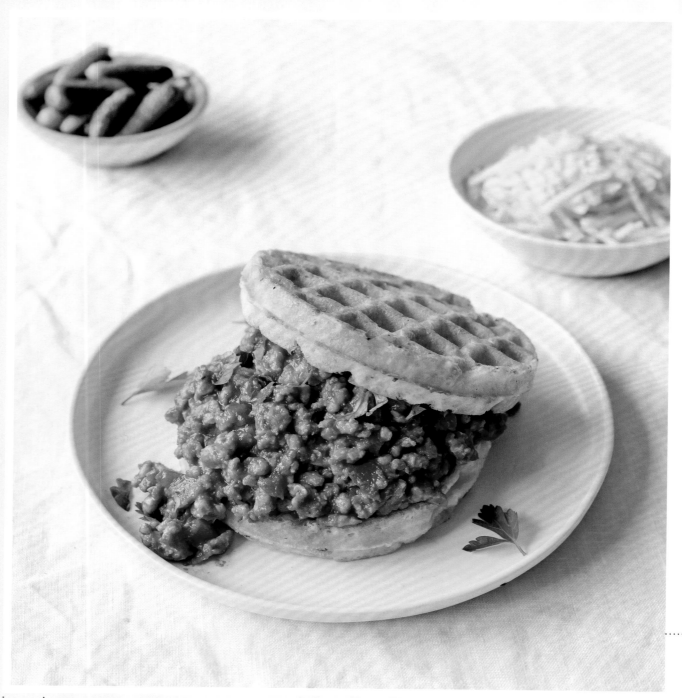

Sweet and Savory Keto Chaffles

Servings:
2 chaffle stacks

Hands-on time:
15 minutes

Overall time:
20 minutes

Chaffle Sloppy Joes

A healthier take on an American classic. These Sloppy Joes are messy, saucy, and just as delicious—but with just a fraction of the carbs.

INGREDIENTS

2 Basic Savory Chaffles (page 14)

8.8 ounces (250 g) ground turkey

1 tablespoon (15 ml) ghee or duck fat

1 teaspoon onion powder

¼ teaspoon garlic powder

½ medium (60 g/2.1 oz) red bell pepper, finely diced

¼ teaspoon chili powder

½ teaspoon Dijon mustard

1½ teaspoons coconut aminos

1 tablespoon (15 ml) tomato paste

⅓ cup (80 g/2.8 oz) canned tomatoes, ideally peeled

Salt and pepper, to taste

1 tablespoon (3 g/0.2 oz) chopped fresh chives, parsley, or spring onion

INSTRUCTIONS

To make the chaffles, follow the instructions for the Basic Chaffles on page 14. When the chaffles are done, set aside.

Place the turkey on a hot pan greased with ghee and cook over medium-high heat for 5 to 7 minutes, or until opaque. Use a slotted spoon to transfer the browned meat to a plate and set aside. Add the onion powder, garlic powder, bell pepper, chili powder, Dijon mustard, coconut aminos, tomato paste, and tomatoes. Stir to combine. Bring to a boil and cook for 5 minutes, or until the pepper is crisp and tender. Season with salt and pepper to taste and take it off the heat.

To assemble, top the chaffles with the cooked turkey and sprinkle with herbs. Serve warm. The turkey topping can be stored in a sealed jar in the fridge for up to 4 days. Reheat before serving.

TIP

* For an even more satisfying meal, you can serve this as a sandwich. To do that, you'll need an extra two chaffles (one for each serving).

Nutrition facts (1 chaffle stack, served with 1 chaffle)

Total carbs:	Fiber:	Net carbs:	Protein:	Fat:	Calories:	Calories from
9.2 g	**3.2 g**	**6 g**	**34.5 g**	**41.9 g**	**545 kcal**	**carbs (4%) protein (26%) fat (70%)**

Servings:
2 chaffle stacks

Hands-on time:
20 minutes

Overall time:
25 minutes

Buffalo Chicken Chaffle Stacks

This is a hearty sandwich that will please those who love Buffalo chicken wings. It is even better when you can pair it with a simple cabbage-and-celery slaw covered in homemade blue cheese dressing!

INGREDIENTS

2 Basic Savory Chaffles (page 14)

Slaw with Blue Cheese Dressing

2 tablespoons (30 ml) mayonnaise made from healthy fats such as avocado oil

2 tablespoons (15 g/0.5 oz) crumbled blue cheese

¼ teaspoon onion powder

2 teaspoons (10 ml) fresh lemon juice

⅛ teaspoon dried celery seeds

1 small (40 g/1.4 oz) celery stick, thinly sliced

1 cup (70 g/2.5 oz) shredded white cabbage or prepared coleslaw mix (no dressing)

Salt and pepper, to taste

Chicken Patties

8.8 ounces (250 g) ground chicken or turkey

1 tablespoon (15 ml) hot sauce (buffalo sauce or Sriracha), plus more for serving

¼ teaspoon salt

Pinch of black pepper

2 tablespoons (8 g/0.3 oz) chopped fresh parsley, plus more for serving

2 teaspoons (10 ml) ghee or duck fat for frying

Nutrition facts (1 chaffle stack + ½ slaw, served with 1 chaffle)

Total carbs:	Fiber:	Net carbs:	Protein:	Fat:	Calories:	Calories from
8.1 g	**2.8 g**	**5.3 g**	**41.5 g**	**36.8 g**	**528 kcal**	**carbs (4%)** **protein (32%)** **fat (64%)**

INSTRUCTIONS

To cook the batter, follow the instructions for the Basic Chaffles on page 14. When the chaffles are done, set aside.

To make the slaw, place the mayonnaise, blue cheese, onion powder, lemon juice, and celery seeds into a medium mixing bowl. Add the celery and cabbage. Toss to combine. Season with salt and pepper to taste. Cover and refrigerate until ready to be used.

To make the patties, place all of the ingredients in a bowl and combine using your hands. Alternatively, place all of the ingredients apart from the parsley in a food processor and pulse until well combined. Then stir in the parsley. Divide the meat into 2 equal parts (about 137 g/ 4.8 oz each). Use your hands to shape each part into a patty, about 3 inches (9 cm) in diameter and ½ to ¾ inch (1¼ to 2 cm) thick.

Heat a large pan greased with the ghee over medium-high heat. Use a spatula to transfer the patties to the hot pan. Cook for 3 to 4 minutes, and then flip over with the spatula and cook for an additional 3 to 4 minutes. Set aside.

To assemble, top the chaffles with chicken patties. Top with the slaw or serve it as a side. Optionally, serve with more parsley and hot sauce. The patties and slaw can be stored in separate sealed jars in the fridge for up to 3 days. Reheat the patties before serving.

TIP

* For an even more satisfying meal, you can serve this as a sandwich. To do that, you'll need an extra two chaffles (one for each serving).

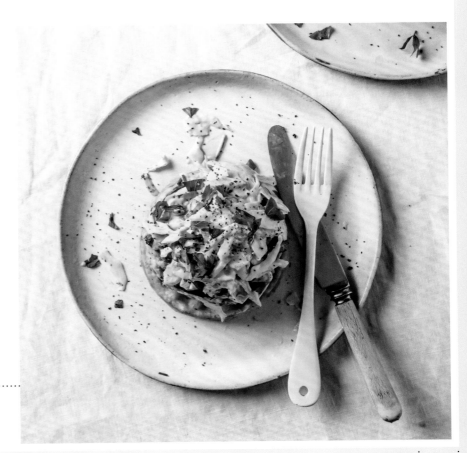

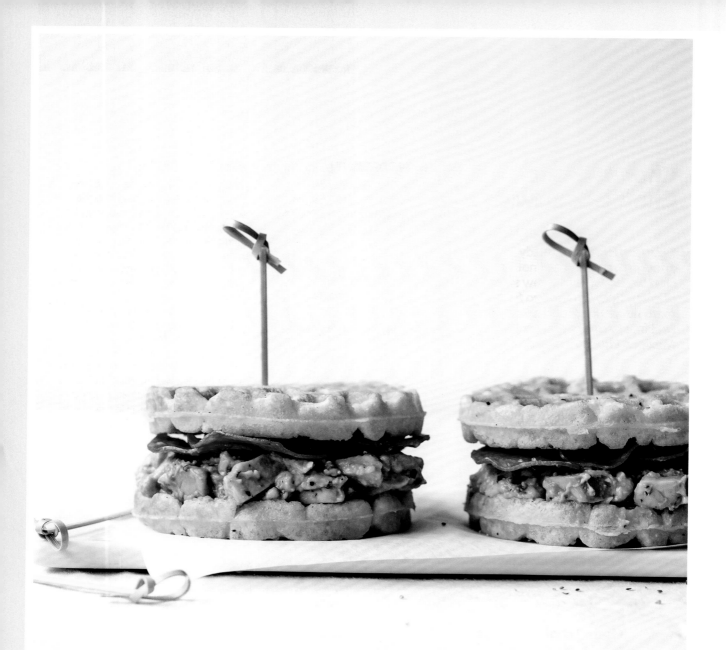

Servings:
2 chaffle sandwiches

Hands-on time:
15 minutes

Overall time:
20 minutes

Chorizo Guac Chaffle Sandwich

If guacamole isn't already enough to make your mouth start watering, add a few slices of crispy Spanish chorizo for an extra flavor boost and spicy kick. Feel free to use crisp crumbled Mexican chorizo instead.

INGREDIENTS

Quick Guacamole
1 small (100 g/3.5 oz) ripe avocado, peeled and pitted

1 tablespoon (15 ml) fresh lime juice

2 tablespoons (14 g/0.5 oz) diced yellow onion

1 teaspoon chopped red chile pepper

½ teaspoon minced garlic (½ clove)

4 or 5 cherry tomatoes, chopped (40 g/1.4 oz)

1 tablespoon (4 g/0.2 oz) chopped fresh cilantro or parsley

Salt and pepper, to taste

Chaffles
4 Basic Savory Chaffles (page 14)

8–10 slices (30 g/1.1 oz) Spanish chorizo or pepperoni

INSTRUCTIONS

Place half of the avocado into a bowl and mash well with a fork. Add the lime juice, onion, chile pepper, garlic, and tomatoes. Stir to combine. Dice the remaining avocado and mix it in, but do not mash it. Add the cilantro, and season with salt and black pepper to taste. Cover and refrigerate until ready to serve.

To crisp up the chorizo, place the slices in a hot dry pan and let them cook for 1 to 2 minutes.

To assemble, top the chaffles with the guacamole. Add the crispy chorizo slices and top with another chaffle. The guacamole is best eaten within a day, but it can be stored in a separate sealed container in the fridge for up to 3 days.

Nutrition facts (1 chaffle sandwich)

Total carbs:	Fiber:	Net carbs:	Protein:	Fat:	Calories:	Calories from
13.8 g	**6.5 g**	**7.3 g**	**29.5 g**	**50 g**	**608 kcal**	**carbs (5%) protein (20%) fat (75%)**

Servings:
1 chaffle sandwich

Hands-on time:
10 minutes

Overall time:
15 minutes

Reuben Sandwich Chaffle Panini

I've always loved sandwiches that have more filling than they have bread—just like this Reuben. Serve half a sandwich for a light meal or the whole sandwich for a complete meal. Chaffle sandwiches are more filling than you think!

INGREDIENTS

Chaffles
2 Basic Savory Chaffles using Swiss cheese (page 14)

4 slices (60 g/2.1 oz) pastrami

2 slices (40 g/1.6 oz) Swiss cheese

¼ cup (36 g/1.3 oz) drained sauerkraut

Russian Dressing
1½ tablespoons (23 ml) mayonnaise made from healthy fats such as avocado oil

½ teaspoon Sriracha sauce

1 teaspoon fresh lemon juice

1 teaspoon grated pickles

¼ teaspoon prepared horseradish

1 small (10 g/0.4 oz) spring onion, chopped

Salt and pepper, to taste

INSTRUCTIONS

To make the chaffles, follow the instructions for the Basic Chaffles on page 14. You can use a mini waffle maker with a waffle or a panini grid—either will work. When the chaffles are done, set aside.

To make the dressing, combine the mayonnaise, Sriracha, lemon juice, pickles, horseradish, spring onion, salt, and pepper in a small bowl. Set aside.

To assemble, top one chaffle with slices of pastrami, cheese, and sauerkraut. Finally, drizzle with the dressing and top with the remaining chaffle. Serve warm.

TIP

* For the most authentic Reuben sandwich, swap the basic chaffle for the Rye Bread Chaffles (page 20)!

* If a full serving is too much for you, serve half of the sandwich alongside any salad.

Nutrition facts (1 chaffle sandwich)

Total carbs:	Fiber:	Net carbs:	Protein:	Fat:	Calories	Calories from
8.7 g	**3.9 g**	**4.8 g**	**46.6 g**	**61.4 g**	**772 kcal**	**carbs (2%)** **protein (24%)** **fat (74%)**

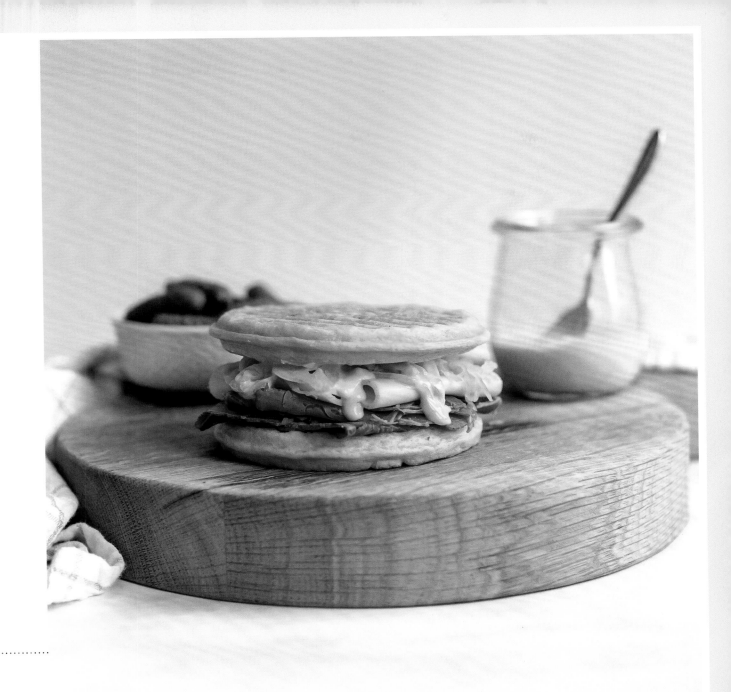

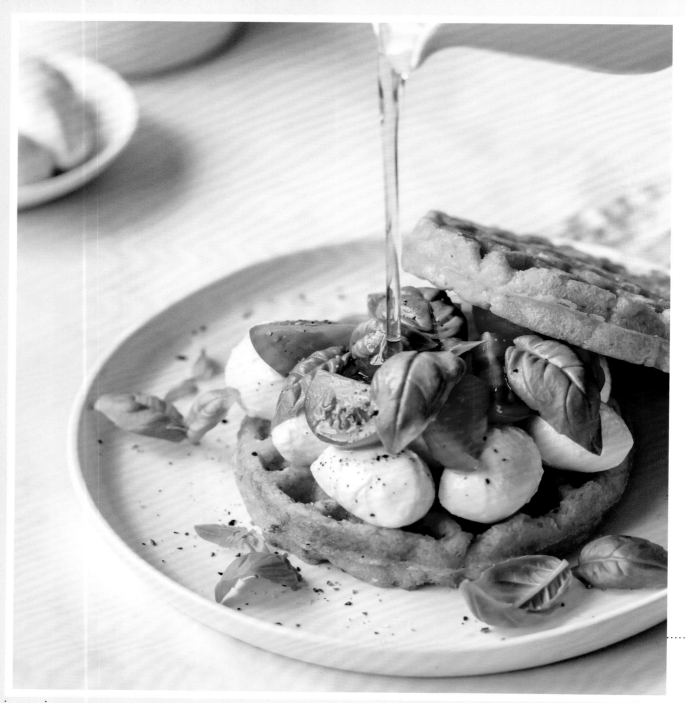

Servings:
1 chaffle sandwich

Hands-on time:
10 minutes

Overall time:
15 minutes

Tricolore Chaffle Sandwich

This recipe is inspired by a traditional Mediterranean salad. It features the colors and flavors of Italy in one easy chaffle sandwich!

INGREDIENTS

Chaffles
Ingredients for 2 Basic Savory Chaffles, ideally made with shredded mozzarella (page 14)

1 tablespoon (15 ml) red or green pesto (Pesto 2 Ways, page 11)

Topping
2 ounces mini fresh mozzarella balls or sliced fresh mozzarella (57 g)

2 or 3 cherry tomatoes (15 g/0.5 oz), quartered

A few fresh basil leaves

Pinch of black pepper

1 teaspoon extra-virgin olive oil

INSTRUCTIONS

Follow the instructions for the Basic Savory Chaffles on page 14. Make two chaffles, adding pesto to the batter. This recipe yields slightly more batter, so it's better if you add it gradually in two parts per chaffle to avoid overflowing (see leakproof tips, page 8). Close and cook until crisp just like any chaffle. Let it cool down before topping.

Top the chaffles with fresh mozzarella, tomatoes, and basil. Sprinkle with black pepper and drizzle olive oil on top. Top with the second chaffle and serve immediately.

TIP

* Want to make a lighter dish? Skip the top chaffle and serve as a stack instead of a sandwich, with just 1 chaffle plus the topping.

Nutrition facts (1 chaffle sandwich)

Total carbs:	Fiber:	Net carbs:	Protein:	Fat:	Calories:	Calories from
12.2 g	**3.2 g**	**9 g**	**39.6 g**	**48.8 g**	**636 kcal**	**carbs (6%)** **protein (25%)** **fat (69%)**

Servings:
1 chaffle sandwich

Hands-on time:
10 minutes

Overall time:
15 minutes

Avocado & Egg Chaffle Sandwich

This grab-n-go sandwich may just become your weekly staple. Eggs contain the highest quality protein, and avocados will fuel your body with healthy monounsaturated fats and potassium. So good for you!

INGREDIENTS

2 Basic Savory Chaffles (page 14)

2 large eggs, hard-boiled, or use 1½ hard-boiled duck eggs

1½ tablespoons (23 ml) mayonnaise made from healthy fats such as avocado oil

¼ teaspoon Dijon mustard

Salt and pepper, to taste

1 medium (15 g/0.5 oz) spring onion, sliced

½ small (50 g/1.8 oz) avocado, peeled, pitted, and sliced

INSTRUCTIONS

To make the chaffles, follow the instructions for the Basic Chaffles on page 14. You can use a mini waffle maker with a waffle or a panini grid—either will work. When the chaffles are done, set aside.

Peel and dice the eggs and place in a bowl. Add the mayonnaise and Dijon mustard, and season with salt and pepper to taste. Add the spring onion and stir until well combined.

To assemble, top one chaffle with the avocado salad and then add the avocado (or you can mix avocado into the egg salad) and the remaining chaffle. Serve warm.

Nutrition facts (1 chaffle sandwich)

Total carbs:	Fiber:	Net carbs:	Protein:	Fat:	Calories:	Calories from
13.4 g	**6.3 g**	**7.1 g**	**38.7 g**	**72.3 g**	**844 kcal**	**carbs (3%)** **protein (19%)** **fat (78%)**

TIP

* **Hard-boiled eggs:** Fresh eggs don't peel well. It's better if you use eggs that you bought 7 to 10 days before cooking. Place the eggs in a pot and fill with water, covering them by an inch (2.5 cm). Bring to a boil over high heat. Turn off the heat and cover with a lid. Remove from the burner and keep the eggs covered in the pot (10 to 12 minutes for medium-sized eggs; 13 to 14 minutes for large; 15 to 16 minutes for extra-large; 17 to 18 minutes for jumbo and duck eggs). When done, transfer to a bowl filled with ice water and let the eggs sit for 5 minutes. To peel, remove from the ice water and knock each egg several times against the countertop or work surface to crack the shells. Gently peel off the shells. Once cooled, store unpeeled in the fridge for up to 1 week.

* If a full serving is too much for you, serve half of the sandwich alongside any salad.

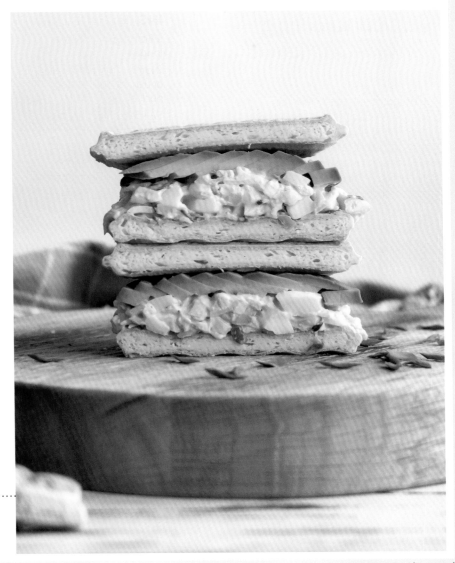

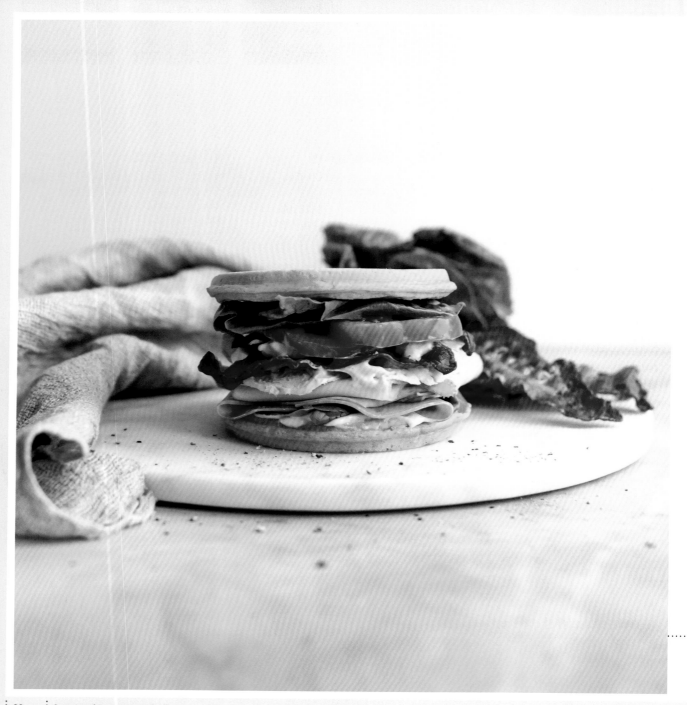

Servings:
1 chaffle sandwich

Hands-on time:
10 minutes

Overall time:
15 minutes

Club Chaffle Sandwich

These chaffles are inspired by the clubhouse sandwich, one of the most iconic sandwiches on the menu of any snack bar. And it's no wonder—all those delicious layers of ham, cheese, chicken, bacon, tomato, and lettuce create the perfect moreish bite.

INGREDIENTS

2 Basic Savory Chaffles (page 14)

1½ tablespoons (23 ml) mayonnaise made from healthy fats such as avocado oil

2 lettuce leaves (15 g/0.5 oz)

2 slices (50 g/1.8 oz) ham

2 slices (40 g/1.4 oz) cheddar cheese

2 slices (40 g/1.4 oz) cooked chicken or turkey

2 thin-cut slices (30 g/1.1 oz) bacon, crisp

2 slices (40 g/1.4 oz) medium tomato

INSTRUCTIONS

To make the chaffles, follow the instructions for the Basic Chaffles on page 14. You can use a mini waffle maker with a waffle or a panini grid—either will work. When the chaffles are done, set aside.

Place the bacon in a hot pan and add a tablespoon (15 ml) of water. Cook over medium-low heat for a few minutes, until the bacon grease is rendered, and cook for 1 to 2 more minutes to crisp up. Then take it off the heat.

To assemble, spread half of the mayonnaise on one chaffle. Add half of the lettuce, slices of ham, cheese, chicken, bacon, the remaining mayonnaise, and tomato slices. Top with the other chaffle. Serve.

TIP

✳ If a full serving is too much for you, serve half of the sandwich alongside any salad.

Nutrition facts (1 chaffle sandwich)

Total carbs:	Fiber:	Net carbs:	Protein:	Fat:	Calories:	Calories from
10.5 g	**3.1 g**	**7.4 g**	**59.3 g**	**67.1 g**	**875 kcal**	**carbs (3%) protein (27%) fat (70%)**

Servings:
1 chaffle sandwich

Hands-on time:
10 minutes

Overall time:
15 minutes

Tuna Melt Chaffle Sandwich

Meet the ultimate tuna melt chaffle! This sandwich takes just a few minutes to assemble and tastes like the real deal. You will never feel like you're missing out on anything.

INGREDIENTS

2 Basic Savory Chaffles (page 14)

½ cup (77 g/2.7 oz) canned tuna, drained

1½ tablespoons (23 ml) mayonnaise made from healthy fats such as avocado oil

1 teaspoon fresh lemon juice

¼ teaspoon Dijon mustard

1 small (10 g/0.4 oz) spring onion, chopped

Salt and pepper, to taste

2 slices (40 g/1.4 oz) provolone cheese

INSTRUCTIONS

To make the chaffles, follow the instructions for the Basic Chaffles on page 14. You can use a mini waffle maker with a waffle or a panini grid—either will work. When the chaffles are done, set aside.

In a bowl, combine the tuna, mayonnaise, lemon juice, Dijon mustard, and spring onion. Season with salt and pepper to taste.

To assemble, spoon the tuna filling on top of one chaffle. Top with the slices of cheese. Optionally, place under a broiler for 1 to 2 minutes, until the cheese starts to melt. Top with the other chaffle. Serve.

TIP

✱ If a full serving is too much for you, serve half of the sandwich alongside any salad.

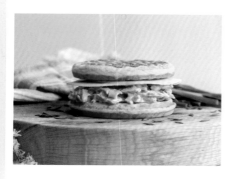

Nutrition facts (1 chaffle sandwich)

Total carbs:	Fiber:	Net carbs:	Protein:	Fat:	Calories:	Calories from
8.8 g	**2.8 g**	**6 g**	**50.2 g**	**66.8 g**	**826 kcal**	**carbs (3%)** **protein (24%)** **fat (73%)**

Monte Cristo Chaffle Sandwich

I'll be honest, I didn't expect this recipe to work and I wasn't sure about using chaffles. They seemed to be too thick and rich for this recipe. That was before I discovered the magic of blending! It produces the fluffiest chaffle that is perfect for making an almost-authentic Monte Cristo sandwich.

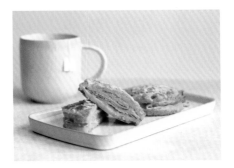

INGREDIENTS

2 Basic Savory Chaffles (page 14)

4 teaspoons (20 ml) mayonnaise made from healthy fats such as avocado oil

1 teaspoon Dijon mustard or 1 tablespoon (15 ml) yellow mustard

½ cup (57 g/2 oz) grated Swiss cheese

3 slices (60 g/2.1 oz) ham

1 large egg

Pinch each of salt and pepper

1 teaspoon ghee or duck fat for frying

Optional: powdered low-carb sweetener such as erythritol, or maple-flavored low-carb syrup

INSTRUCTIONS

To make the chaffles, follow the instructions for the Basic Chaffles on page 14. You can use a mini waffle maker with a waffle or a panini grid—either will work. When the chaffles are done, set aside to cool down slightly; do not let them get too crispy. Using a sharp knife, carefully cut the chaffles widthwise.

Spread 1 teaspoon of mayonnaise and ¼ teaspoon Dijon mustard on the cut side of each chaffle. Layer a sprinkle of the cheese on top of two chaffles, followed by ham and another sprinkle of the cheese. Top with the remaining chaffles to get a total of 2 sandwiches.

Beat the egg and a pinch of salt and pepper. Dip each sandwich in the beaten egg and fry on a hot pan greased with ghee over medium heat. Cook for 2 to 3 minutes per side, until the cheese has melted and the sandwich is crisp to your liking. If you have any cheese left, sprinkle it on top of the sandwiches after you turn them and let it melt as the sandwiches cook.

To serve, slice and optionally serve with a dusting of powdered low-carb sweetener.

Nutrition facts (1 chaffle sandwich)

Total carbs:	Fiber:	Net carbs:	Protein:	Fat:	Calories:	Calories from
4.2 g	**1.3 g**	**2.9 g**	**29.2 g**	**41.1 g**	**500 kcal**	**carbs (2%) protein (23%) fat (75%)**

Lasagna Chaffle Bake

Chaffles are versatile! Imagine chaffles topped with saucy marinara beef, creamy ricotta, and melty mozzarella. It's like a cross between a deep-dish pizza and your favorite Italian casserole.

INGREDIENTS

Chaffles (Triple Batch of Basic Savory Chaffles)

3 large eggs

1½ cups (170 g/6 oz) grated mozzarella

¾ cup (75 g/2.7 oz) almond flour

¾ teaspoon gluten-free baking powder

Filling

1 teaspoon ghee, olive oil, or duck fat

1.1 pounds (500 g) ground beef

¾ cup (180 ml) Marinara Sauce (page 10)

1 cup (240 g/8.5 oz) ricotta cheese

2 tablespoons (8 g/0.3 oz) chopped fresh herbs such as basil, parsley, and mint

1 large egg yolk

½ teaspoon salt

¼ teaspoon black pepper

½ cup (45 g/1.6 oz) Parmesan cheese

½ cup (57 g/2 oz) grated mozzarella cheese

½ cup (57 g/2 oz) grated Emmental or more mozzarella cheese

Nutrition facts (1 chaffle slice)

Total carbs:	Fiber:	Net carbs:	Protein:	Fat:	Calories:	Calories from
8.3 g	**1.7 g**	**6.6 g**	**39.7 g**	**49.9 g**	**641 kcal**	**carbs (4%)** **protein (25%)** **fat (71%)**

INSTRUCTIONS

To make the chaffles, follow the instructions for the Basic Savory Chaffles on page 14, but use a square 5-inch (12.5-cm) Belgian waffle maker instead to make a total of 5 regular-sized (5-inch/12.5-cm) Belgian square chaffles. Preheat the waffle maker. Mix or preferably blend the eggs, mozzarella, almond flour, and baking powder. Spoon about ⅓ cup (80 g/2.8 oz) of the batter into each square of the hot waffle maker. Close the waffle maker and cook for about 3 minutes. Keep an eye on the batter in case it overflows (see leakproof tips on page 8). When done, open the lid and let cool down for a few seconds. Use a spatula to gently transfer the chaffle onto a cooling rack. Repeat for the remaining batter.

To make the beef filling, place the beef in a hot pan greased with ghee. Cook over medium-high heat for about 5 minutes, or until opaque. Stir in the Marinara Sauce and cook for 2 to 3 minutes. Take it off the heat.

Preheat the oven to 350°F (175°C) fan assisted or 380°F (195°C, or gas mark 5½) conventional. In a bowl, mix the ricotta, herbs, egg yolk, salt, and pepper. Set aside.

Use a baking tray or a casserole dish large enough to fit the chaffles in a single layer. Place the chaffles in the tray (cut the fifth chaffle in half for a square shape) and top with the ricotta cheese mixture, cooked beef, and the two types of cheese. Place in the oven and bake for 20 to 25 minutes, or until the cheese has melted and is crisp. Slice into 6 equal pieces. Serve warm or let it cool down and refrigerate for up to 4 days. Reheat before serving.

TIPS

* Thinner slices of chaffles will result in a more pasta-like effect—simply use 2½ Belgian square chaffles and cut them in half widthwise (instead of using 5 square waffles).

* For this recipe, a Belgian square waffle maker works better than round one, but you could use a round mini waffle maker to make more smaller waffles.

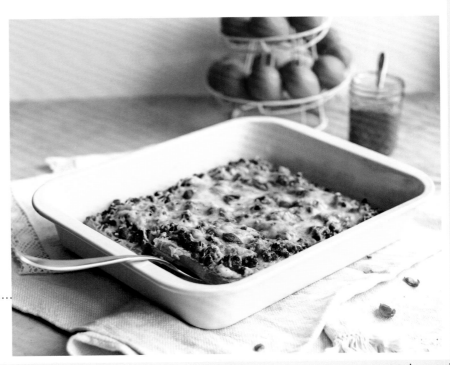

Chapter 4

Sweet Chaffles

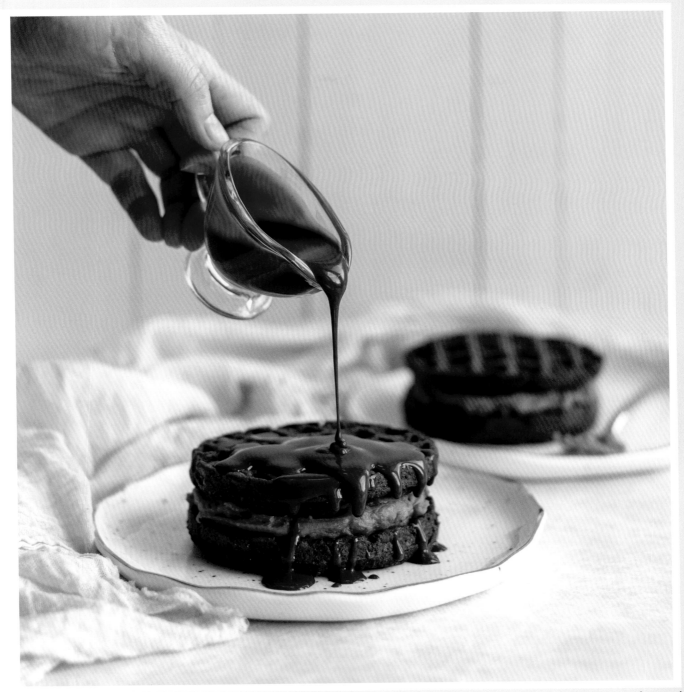

Fluffy Sweet Chaffles Two Ways

Want to make the fluffiest chaffles? I think it's time I introduce you to the best way to make light and fluffy chaffles. This is the perfect combination for light desserts such as Triple Chocolate Chaffle Cake (page 152).

INGREDIENTS

White Chaffles

1 large egg

1 large egg white

2 tablespoons (30 g/1.1 oz) cream cheese

½ cup (57 g/2 oz) grated mozzarella

¼ cup (25 g/0.9 oz) almond flour

2 tablespoons (16 g/0.6 oz) coconut flour

¼ cup (40 g/1.4 oz) granulated low-carb sweetener such as erythritol or Swerve

½ teaspoon gluten-free baking powder

Optional: ¼ to ½ teaspoon sugar-free vanilla extract, pinch of vanilla powder, or pinch of cinnamon

Chocolate Chaffles

1 large egg

1 large egg white

2 tablespoons (30 g/1.1 oz) cream cheese

½ cup (57 g/2 oz) grated mozzarella

2 tablespoons (11 g/0.4 oz) cacao powder

2 tablespoons (16 g/0.6 oz) coconut flour

¼ cup (40 g/1.4 oz) granulated low-carb sweetener such as erythritol or Swerve

½ teaspoon gluten-free baking powder

Nutrition facts (1 white chaffle/1 chocolate chaffle)

Total carbs:	Fiber:	Net carbs:	Protein:	Fat:	Calories:	Calories from
4.1/4.5 g	**1.3/1.7 g**	**2.8/2.8 g**	**8.4/7.6 g**	**10/7.1 g**	**136/106 kcal**	**carbs (8/11%)** **protein (25/29%)** **fat (67/60%)**

INSTRUCTIONS

Preheat the mini waffle maker. Place the egg, egg white, cream cheese, and mozzarella into a blender. (Remember, making truly fluffy chaffles requires blending!) Process until smooth. Add the remaining ingredients and process again.

Spoon one-quarter of the batter into the hot waffle maker (about 65 g/2.3 oz for white chaffles, and 62 g/2.2 oz for chocolate chaffles). Close the waffle maker and cook for 2 to 4 minutes, checking the waffles after 2 minutes.

Keep an eye on the batter in case it overflows (see leakproof tips on page 8). When the chaffles are done, open the lid and let cool down for a few seconds. Use a spatula to gently transfer the chaffle onto a cooling rack. Repeat for the remaining batter. The chaffles will be soft when they are warm, but they will crisp up as they cool down completely.

Enjoy immediately or store in a sealed container at room temperature for up to 1 day, or in the fridge for up to 1 week. The container will keep them soft, but you can leave them uncovered if you prefer them crispy.

TIP

✻ How to make thinner chaffles: Instead of 4 mini fluffy chaffles, some recipes will ask you to make 6 thinner chaffles (about 43 g/1.5 oz of batter for white chaffles, and 41 g/1.4 oz for chocolate chaffles), or up to 8 super thin chaffles (about 32 g/1.1 oz of batter for white chaffles, and 31 g/1.1 oz for chocolate chaffles). Use the back of a spoon or a rubber spatula to spread the batter all over the waffle iron. Keep an eye on the thinner chaffles, as thinner chaffles take just 30 to 90 seconds to cook and can burn easily. Instead of making thinner chaffles, you can also cut the thicker chaffles widthwise. To do that, make sure they are still warm, as it's hard to cut them as they crisp up.

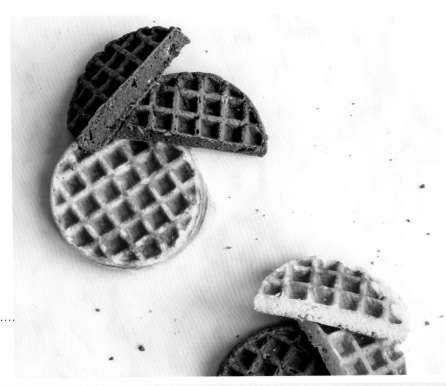

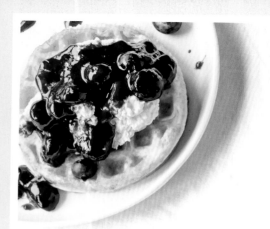

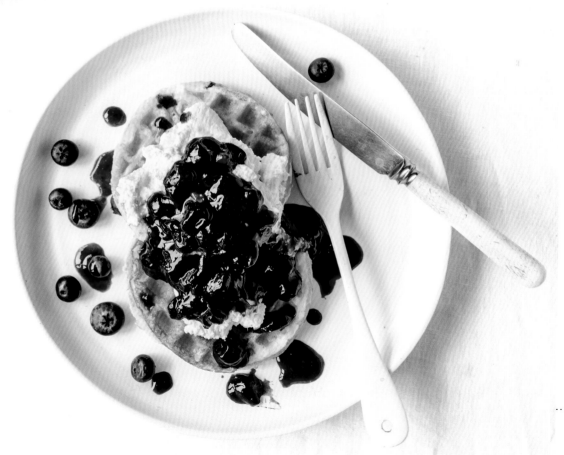

Servings:
3 mini chaffles

Hands-on time:
10 minutes

Overall time:
15 minutes

Breakfast Pancake Chaffles

These chaffles are served just like your breakfast pancakes, with soft and pillowy whipped cream topped with sweet blueberry sauce. A tasty way to start your day!

INGREDIENTS

3 Basic Sweet Chaffles (page 14)

⅔ cup (100 g/3.5 oz) fresh or frozen wild blueberries

Optional: ¼ teaspoon xanthan gum or 1 tablespoon (8 g/ 0.3 oz) chia seeds to thicken

Optional: 1 tablespoon (10 g/ 0.4 oz) granulated low-carb sweetener such as erythritol or Swerve, or to taste

⅔ cup (160 ml) heavy whipping cream, whipped

INSTRUCTIONS

Prepare a batch of the Basic Sweet Chaffles by following the instructions on page 14. When the chaffles are done, let them cool down slightly.

To make the berry sauce, place the blueberries and 2 tablespoons (30 ml) water in a saucepan and bring to a boil. Cook for 3 to 5 minutes, until the berries release their juices. Optionally, add sweetener and stir in. Set aside.

Sprinkle the xanthan gum or chia seeds on top (if using) and mix to combine. If using chia seeds, let them soak for 15 to 20 minutes.

Serve the chaffles with whipped cream and blueberry sauce on top and eat immediately. The berry sauce can be stored in the fridge in a sealed jar for up to 5 days.

TIP

✱ Swap the blueberries for raspberries, strawberries, or blackberries!

Nutrition facts (1 chaffle + about 4 tablespoons whipped cream + 2 tablespoons berry sauce)

Total carbs:	Fiber:	Net carbs:	Protein:	Fat:	Calories:	Calories from
8.8 g	**1.7 g**	**7.1 g**	**9.8 g**	**30.2 g**	**346 kcal**	**carbs (8%) protein (12%) fat (80%)**

Servings:
3 mini chaffles

Hands-on time:
10 minutes

Overall time:
15 minutes

Snickerdoodle Chaffles

These chaffles are like a cross between snickerdoodle cookies and churros. They are soft inside and crispy on the outside with crunchy cinnamon coating. Feel free to serve with soft and fluffy whipped cream.

INGREDIENTS

3 mini Basic Sweet Chaffles (page 14)

1½ tablespoons (23 ml) melted butter or ghee

1 teaspoon cinnamon

3 tablespoons (30 g/1.1 oz) granulated low-carb sweetener such as erythritol or Swerve, or to taste

INSTRUCTIONS

Follow the instructions for the Basic Sweet Chaffles on page 14. When the chaffles have cooled down, brush them with butter on all sides.

Mix the cinnamon and granulated low-carb sweetener. Sprinkle over the chaffles. Turn each chaffle to the other side and sprinkle more. Take each chaffle and roll the edges in the leftover sweetener and cinnamon mixture so it's completely covered.

Enjoy immediately or store in a sealed container at room temperature for up to 1 day, or in the fridge for up to 1 week.

TIP

✱ If you prefer a more churro-like shape and texture, use a regular square-shaped waffle maker to make two chaffles, slice them (just like in the Apple Pie Chaffle Dippers, page 114), and fry them before coating in the cinnamon-sweetener mixture (just like in Chaffle Donuts, page 117).

Nutrition facts (1 chaffle)

Total carbs:	Fiber:	Net carbs:	Protein:	Fat:	Calories:	Calories from
4.5 g	**1.3 g**	**3.2 g**	**8.4 g**	**15.5 g**	**186 kcal**	**carbs (7%)** **protein (18%)** **fat (75%)**

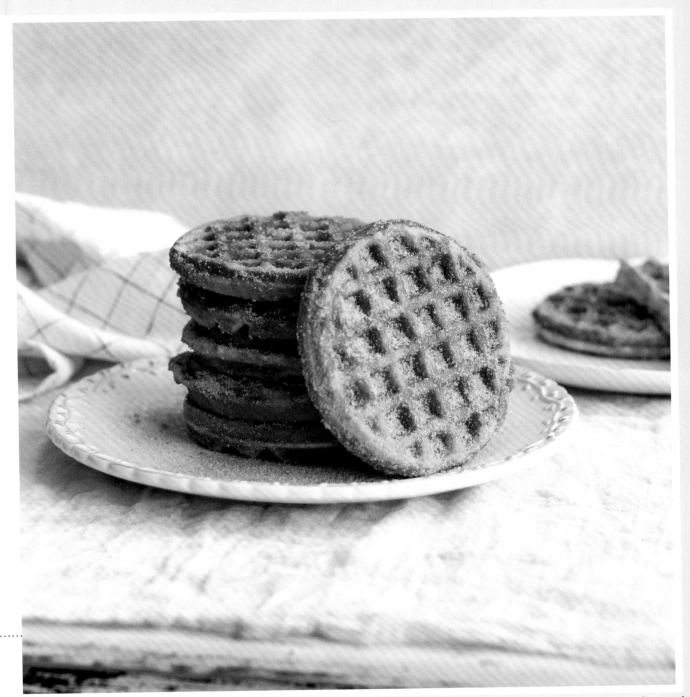

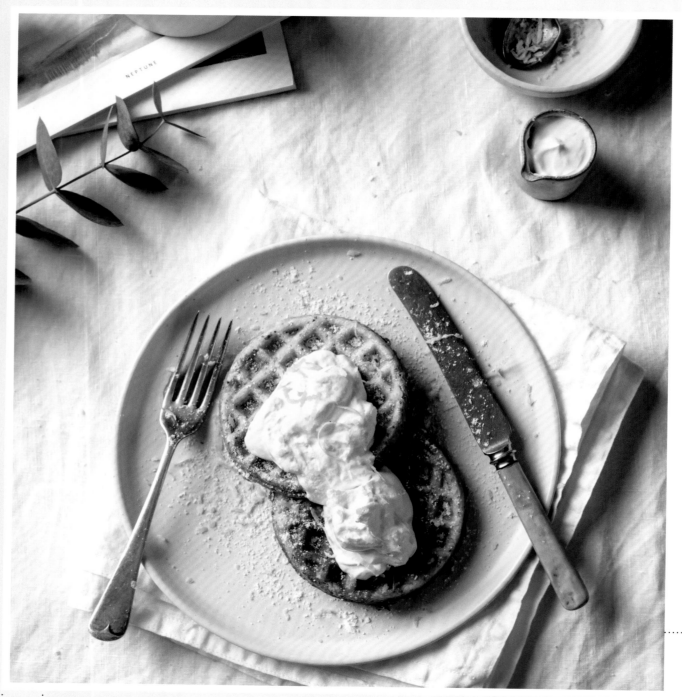

Sweet and Savory Keto Chaffles

Servings:
3 mini chaffles

Hands-on time:
10 minutes

Overall time:
15 minutes

Lemon Poppy Seed Chaffles

These zesty chaffles are like your bakery-style lemon poppy seed muffins. Add lemon-flavored whipped cream on top and you've got the perfect dessert for breakfast!

INGREDIENTS

Chaffles
Ingredients for 3 Basic Sweet Chaffles (page 14)

½ teaspoon fresh lemon zest

1 teaspoon poppy seeds

Lemon Cream
⅔ cup (160 ml) heavy whipping cream

¼ teaspoon lemon zest, plus optionally more for serving

Optional: 1 tablespoon (10 g/ 0.4 oz) powdered low-carb sweetener such as erythritol or Swerve, or to taste

INSTRUCTIONS

Prepare a batch of the Basic Sweet Chaffles by following the instructions on page 14, adding lemon zest and poppy seeds to the batter. If you're blending the batter, add the poppy seeds after the blending. When the chaffles are done, let them cool down slightly.

Whip the cream with lemon zest and an optional sweetener. Serve the chaffles topped with whipped cream and more zest (if using) and eat immediately.

TIP

✻ Swap the cream topping for lemon glaze made with 3 tablespoons (45 ml) melted coconut butter, ¼ teaspoon of fresh lemon zest, 1 teaspoon coconut oil, and 1 to 3 teaspoons of powdered erythritol.

Nutrition facts (1 chaffle + about 4 tablespoons whipped cream)

Total carbs:	Fiber:	Net carbs:	Protein:	Fat:	Calories:	Calories from
5 g	**1.1 g**	**3.9 g**	**9.5 g**	**30.3 g**	**331 kcal**	**carbs (5%) protein (12%) fat (83%)**

Roasted Nutty Chaffles

A simple-yet-delicious chaffle recipe and one of my absolute favorites. Roasted nut butter adds an amazing depth of flavor and makes these chaffles soft and fluffy inside and crispy on the outside—you will want to go back for more!

INGREDIENTS

1 large egg

½ cup (57 g/2 oz) grated mozzarella

3 tablespoons (45 g/1.6 oz) roasted almond butter or any roasted nut/seed/coconut butter

1½ tablespoons (12 g/0.4 oz) coconut flour

¼ teaspoon cinnamon or vanilla powder

⅛ teaspoon gluten-free baking powder

3 tablespoons (30 g/1.1 oz) granulated brown sugar substitute, erythritol, or Swerve, or to taste

Optional to serve: dusting of low-carb sweetener, whipped cream, melted dark chocolate, and/or berries

INSTRUCTIONS

Preheat the waffle maker. Blend the egg, mozzarella, nut butter, coconut flour, cinnamon, and baking powder until smooth. Add the sweetener and stir in to combine.

To cook the batter, follow the instructions for the Basic Chaffles on page 14. When filling the waffle maker, use half (about 53 g/1.9 oz) of the batter for each chaffle. Let chaffles cool down. They can be stored just like Basic Chaffles (page 8).

Serve on their own or with a dusting of low-carb sweetener, whipped cream, melted chocolate, and/or berries. Enjoy immediately or store in a sealed container at room temperature for up to 1 day, or in the fridge for up to 1 week. The container will keep them soft, but you can leave them uncovered if you prefer them crispy.

Nutrition facts (1 chaffle)

Total carbs:	Fiber:	Net carbs:	Protein:	Fat:	Calories:	Calories from
6 g	**2.4 g**	**3.6 g**	**10.6 g**	**14.8 g**	**195 kcal**	**carbs (8%)** **protein (22%)** **fat (70%)**

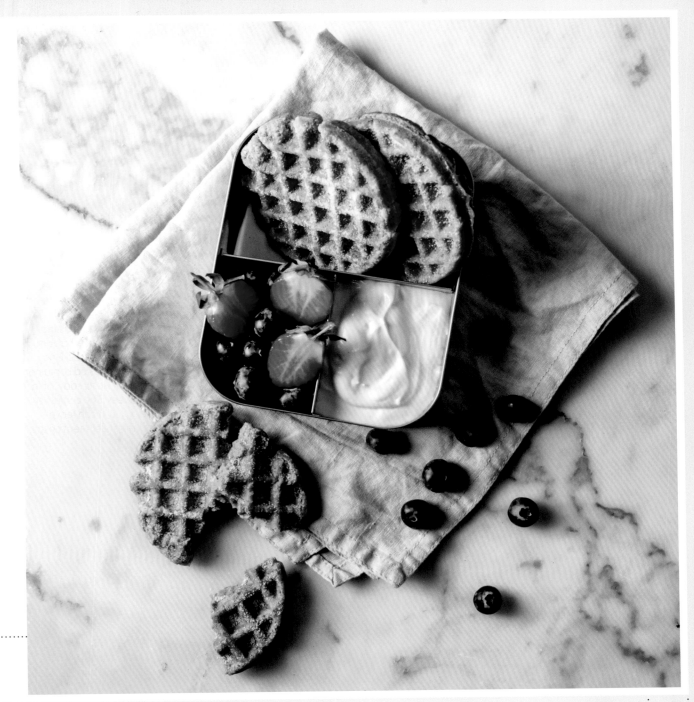

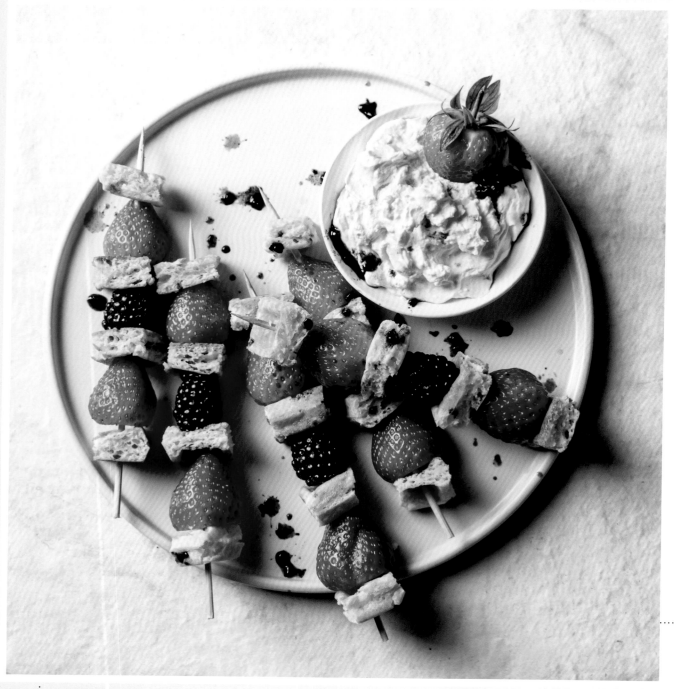

Sweet and Savory Keto Chaffles

Servings:
4 chaffle skewers

Hands-on time:
10 minutes

Overall time:
15 minutes

Chaffle & Berry Skewers

Looking for a super quick yet impressive party snack? Make a few sweet chaffles in advance and keep them in the freezer. Defrost, thread on skewers with berries, and serve with whipped cream—you've got an easy keto dessert in less than 5 minutes!

INGREDIENTS

3 Basic Sweet Chaffles (page 14)

4 large (80 g/2.8 oz) strawberries, halved

4–8 large blackberries or raspberries (40 g/1.4 oz)

⅔ cup (160 ml) heavy whipping cream, whipped, or mascarpone

¼ teaspoon sugar-free vanilla extract

Optional: 1 tablespoon (10 g/ 0.4 oz) powdered low-carb sweetener such as erythritol or Swerve, or to taste

INSTRUCTIONS

Prepare a batch of the Basic Sweet Chaffles by following the instructions on page 14. You can use a regular square 5-inch (12.5-cm) Belgian Waffle maker to make 2 chaffles or a mini waffle maker to make 3 chaffles. When the chaffles are done, let them cool down slightly, and then cut into a total of 12 (for mini chaffles) to 16 (for square chaffles) pieces so you have 3 to 4 pieces per skewer.

Create skewers, each one with chaffle pieces (3 to 4 per chaffle depending on how many you cut), 2 strawberry halves, and a blackberry. Serve with whipped cream or mascarpone mixed with vanilla and optionally low-carb sweetener to taste. Eat immediately or store in the fridge for up to 1 day.

Nutrition facts (1 skewer + about 4 tablespoons whipped cream)

Total carbs:	Fiber:	Net carbs:	Protein:	Fat:	Calories:	Calories from
6 g	**1.6 g**	**4.4 g**	**7.3 g**	**22.6 g**	**256 kcal**	**carbs (7%) protein (12%) fat (81%)**

Servings:
3 mini chaffles

Hands-on time:
10 minutes

Overall time:
15 minutes

Chocolate Chip Cookie Dough Chaffles

Imagine you come home to a plate of freshly baked cookies that smell like the ones your grandma used to make. Then add a scoop of vanilla ice cream. Can you resist? With these keto cookie dough chaffles, you don't have to!

INGREDIENTS

3 Basic Sweet Chaffles (page 14)

1 teaspoon cinnamon

Pinch of salt

½ teaspoon sugar-free vanilla extract

½ teaspoon lemon zest

2 tablespoons (22 g/0.8 oz) 90% dark chocolate chips (85% or more), or sugar-free dark chocolate chips

Optional: serve with No-Churn Vanilla Ice Cream (page 118), whipped cream, coconut cream, or mascarpone

INSTRUCTIONS

Prepare a batch of the Basic Sweet Chaffles by following the instructions on page 14, adding cinnamon, salt, vanilla, and lemon zest to the batter. Blend and then stir in the chocolate chips and spoon in the waffle maker to cook. Keep an eye on the chaffles as the chocolate chips tend to burn. When the chaffles are done, let them cool down slightly.

Eat immediately with optional toppings or store at room temperature for up to 1 day, in the fridge for up to 1 week, or freeze for up to 3 months.

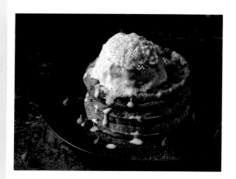

Nutrition facts (1 chaffle)

Total carbs:	Fiber:	Net carbs:	Protein:	Fat:	Calories:	Calories from
5.6 g	**1.8 g**	**3.8 g**	**9.1 g**	**13.9 g**	**177 kcal**	**carbs (9%)** **protein (21%)** **fat (70%)**

Servings:
3 mini chaffles

Hands-on time:
10 minutes

Overall time:
20 minutes

Pumpkin Pie Chaffles

Fancy a slice of pumpkin pie?
These chaffles are a quick-
and-easy breakfast recipe
that can be made with just
a few common ingredients.
The addition of pumpkin
purée makes them soft and
moist inside.

INGREDIENTS

Chaffles
3 Basic Sweet Chaffles
(page 14)

1 tablespoon (20 g/0.7 oz)
pumpkin purée

1 teaspoon (3 g/0.2 oz)
coconut flour

½ teaspoon pumpkin pie spice

Cheesecake Glaze
2 tablespoons (30 g/1.1 oz)
full-fat cream cheese

2 tablespoons (30 ml) heavy
whipping cream

1 tablespoon (10 g/0.4 oz)
powdered low-carb sweetener
such as erythritol or Swerve,
or to taste

¼ teaspoon cinnamon

INSTRUCTIONS

Prepare a batch of the Basic Sweet
Chaffles by following the instructions
on page 14, adding pumpkin purée,
coconut flour, and pumpkin pie spice.
When the chaffles are done, let them
cool down slightly.

To make the cheesecake frosting,
mix together the cream cheese,
whipping cream, sweetener, and
cinnamon. Using a spoon or a piping
bag, add the frosting to the top of
the chaffles.

Eat immediately or store in the
fridge in a sealed container for up to
3 days (with the topping) or up to 1 week
(without the topping), or freeze (without
the cheesecake topping) for up to
3 months.

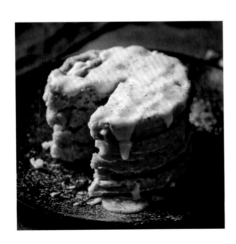

Nutrition facts (1 chaffle + topping)

Total carbs:	Fiber:	Net carbs:	Protein:	Fat:	Calories:	Calories from
5.3 g	**1.5 g**	**3.8 g**	**9.5 g**	**16.5 g**	**200 kcal**	**carbs (8%)** **protein (19%)** **fat (73%)**

Chocolate Marble Chaffles

Want to try something new but only have a few ingredients on hand? Turn your plain chaffles into these cute marble chaffles! Add soft chocolate ganache on top and you'll be in heaven.

INGREDIENTS

Chaffles

3 Basic Sweet Chaffles (page 14)

1 tablespoon (6 g/0.2 oz) cacao powder or Dutch process cocoa powder

Quick Ganache

¼ cup (60 ml) heavy whipping cream

1.2 ounces (35 g) 90% dark chocolate chips (85% or more), or sugar-free dark chocolate chips

Optional: ¼ teaspoon sugar-free vanilla extract and few drops of stevia, to taste

INSTRUCTIONS

Prepare a batch of the Basic Sweet Chaffles by following the instructions on page 14, adding cacao powder. When the chaffles are done, let them cool down slightly.

To make the ganache, heat the cream until hot and then pour into a small bowl over the chocolate chips. Let it sit undisturbed for 1 to 2 minutes and then stir until smooth and glossy. Optionally, mix in vanilla and stevia. Serve on top of the chaffles.

Eat immediately or store in the fridge in a sealed container for up to 5 days or freeze for up to 3 months.

Nutrition facts (1 chaffle + 2 tablespoons ganache)

Total carbs:	Fiber:	Net carbs:	Protein:	Fat:	Calories:	Calories from
7.2 g	**2.3 g**	**4.9 g**	**10.2 g**	**24.1 g**	**274 kcal**	**carbs (7%)** **protein (15%)** **fat (78%)**

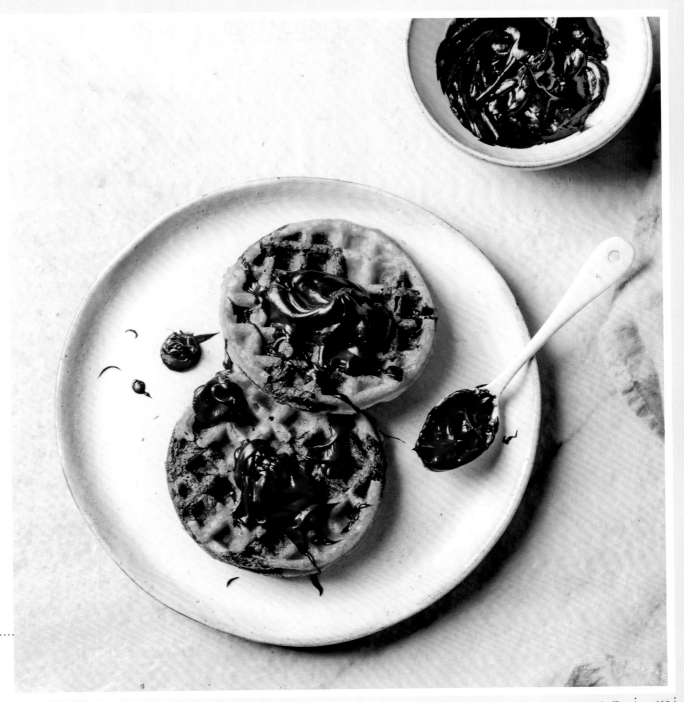

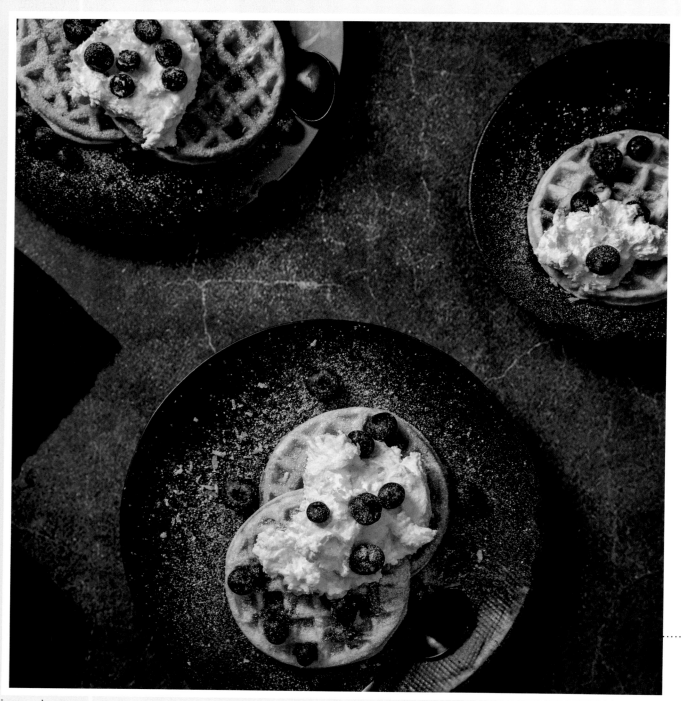

Blueberry Muffin Chaffles

Sometimes the best way is to keep things simple. When I first made these chaffles, I tried adding the blueberries directly into the chaffle batter, but they ended up being too messy and were falling apart. These chaffles are crispy on the outside and soft inside with the perfect balance of sweet blueberries and fluffy cream on top.

INGREDIENTS

3 Basic Sweet Chaffles (page 14, with the optional vanilla extract)

⅔ cup (160 ml) heavy whipping cream

Optional: 1 tablespoon (10 g/ 0.4 oz) powdered low-carb sweetener such as erythritol or Swerve, or to taste

½ cup (75 g/2.7 oz) fresh or frozen wild blueberries

Optional: fresh grated lemon zest or orange zest

INSTRUCTIONS

Prepare a batch of the Basic Sweet Chaffles by following the instructions on page 14. When the chaffles are done, let them cool down slightly.

Whip the cream, optionally with sweetener. Top each chaffle with whipped cream, a few blueberries, and optionally with lemon or orange zest. Serve immediately.

Nutrition facts (1 chaffle + about 4 tablespoons whipped cream + 3 tablespoons blueberries)

Total carbs:	Fiber:	Net carbs:	Protein:	Fat:	Calories:	Calories from
7.7 g	**1.4 g**	**6.3 g**	**9.7 g**	**30.1 g**	**342 kcal**	**carbs (7%) protein (12%) fat (81%)**

Servings:
6 mini chaffles

Hands-on time:
15 minutes

Overall time:
40 minutes

Chocolate Chaffles with Caramelized Pecans

My favorite sweet chaffles of the entire book? You just found them! The candied pecan and dark chocolate layer gives these chaffles an incredibly delicious crunch.

INGREDIENTS

6 Basic Sweet Chaffles (page 14, ideally using brown sugar substitute)

Caramelized Pecans

¾ cup (75 g/2.7 oz) pecans, broken into pieces or chopped roughly

2 teaspoons (10 ml) virgin coconut oil

¼ teaspoon cinnamon

¼ teaspoon vanilla powder or ½ teaspoon sugar-free vanilla extract

1 tablespoon (10 g/0.4 oz) brown sugar substitute or erythritol or Swerve

Pinch of salt

Optional: ½ teaspoon sugar-free maple extract

Chocolate Crust

5 ounces (142 g) 90% dark chocolate chips (85% or more), or sugar-free dark chocolate chips

2 teaspoons (10 ml) virgin coconut oil

INSTRUCTIONS

Prepare a batch of the Basic Sweet Chaffles by following the instructions on page 14. When the chaffles are done, let them cool down completely before adding the topping.

Preheat the oven to 300°F (150°C) fan assisted or 340°F (170°C, or gas mark 3½) conventional. Place the pecans on a baking tray lined with parchment paper. Drizzle with coconut oil and sprinkle with cinnamon, vanilla, sweetener, and salt. Optionally add maple extract. Toss to combine. Place in the oven and bake for 12 to 15 minutes, mixing and tossing once or twice during the baking process. Keep an eye on the nuts, as they tend to burn easily. Once baked, remove from the oven, toss again and let them cool down to room temperature.

Nutrition facts (1 chaffle)

Total carbs:	Fiber:	Net carbs:	Protein:	Fat:	Calories:	Calories from
8.1 g	**3.2 g**	**4.9 g**	**7.7 g**	**30.1 g**	**312 kcal**	**carbs (6%)** **protein (10%)** **fat (84%)**

Meanwhile, melt the dark chocolate with coconut oil and stir to combine. You can use a microwave oven or a double boiler. To use a double boiler, place a bowl over a saucepan filled with about 1 cup (240 ml) water. The bowl should not be touching the surface of the water. Bring to a boil and let it melt. Once melted, let the chocolate cool down to room temperature so it's not too runny.

Spoon about 2 tablespoons (30 ml) of the melted chocolate on top of each chaffle. Top with the caramelized pecans and let the chocolate set completely. Store at room temperature for up to 1 day (uncovered chaffles will crisp up), in a sealed container in the fridge for up to 1 week, or in the freezer for up to 3 months.

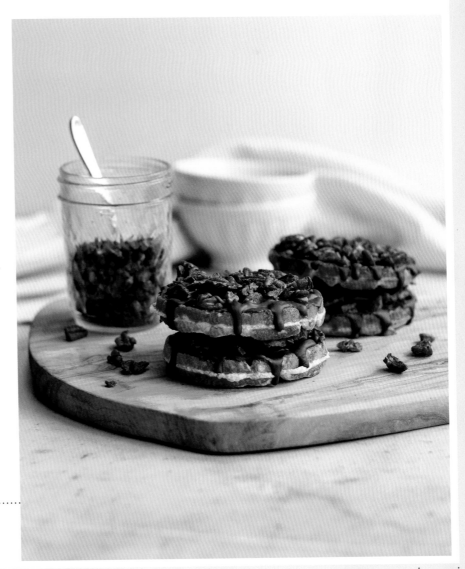

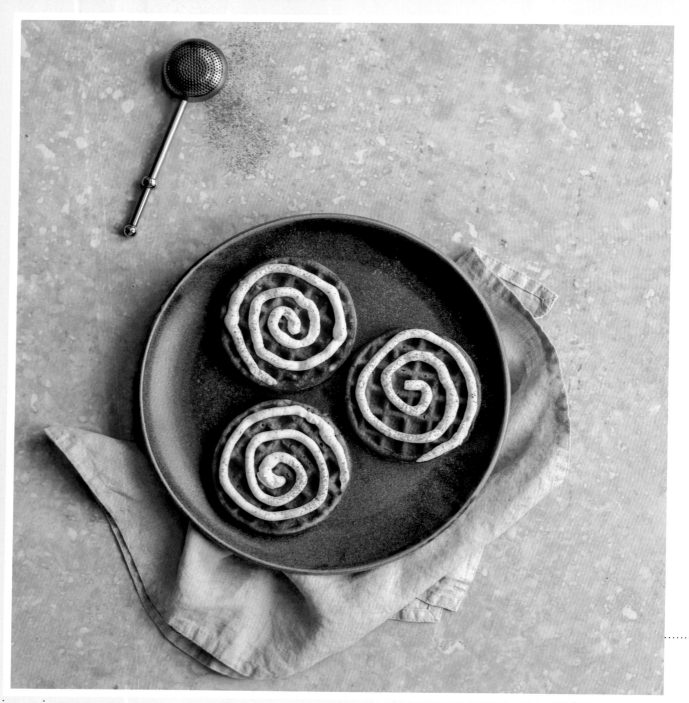

Sweet and Savory Keto Chaffles

Servings:
3 chaffles

Hands-on time:
10 minutes

Overall time:
20 minutes

Cinnamon Roll Chaffles

Are you short on time but craving cinnamon rolls? These waffle iron–style breakfast cinnamon rolls are just what you need to start your day. All of the flavor with none of the hassle or carbs.

INGREDIENTS

Chaffles
3 Basic Sweet Chaffles (page 14)

½ teaspoon cinnamon, plus more for serving

Cheesecake Glaze
2 tablespoons (30 g/1.1 oz) full-fat cream cheese

2 tablespoons (30 ml) heavy whipping cream

1 tablespoon (10 g/0.4 oz) powdered low-carb sweetener such as erythritol or Swerve, or to taste plus more for serving

Pinch of vanilla powder or ¼ teaspoon sugar-free vanilla extract

INSTRUCTIONS

Prepare a batch of the Basic Sweet Chaffles by following the instructions on page 14, adding cinnamon. When the chaffles are done, let them cool down completely.

To make the cheesecake frosting, mix the cream cheese, whipping cream, sweetener, and vanilla. You can simply decorate the chaffles using a spoon, or use a piping bag, to create a spiral effect on top. Dust with more cinnamon and optionally with powdered low-carb sweetener.

Serve immediately or store in the fridge in a sealed container for up to 3 days (with the topping) or up to 1 week (without the topping), or freeze (without the cheesecake topping) for up to 3 months.

Nutrition facts (1 chaffle + topping)

Total carbs:	Fiber:	Net carbs:	Protein:	Fat:	Calories:	Calories from
4.4 g	**1.1 g**	**3.3 g**	**9.3 g**	**16.3 g**	**194 kcal**	**carbs (7%)** **protein (19%)** **fat (74%)**

Servings:
8 chaffle sticks

Hands-on time:
10 minutes

Overall time:
15 minutes

Orange Cardamom Chocolate Chaffle Dippers

There are flavor combinations that just work every single time. Building on the all-time favorite chocolate-and-orange combo, these chaffles are spiced up with fragrant cardamom.

INGREDIENTS

Chaffles

3 Basic Sweet Chaffles (page 14)

1 teaspoon fresh orange zest

⅛ teaspoon ground cardamom, or use ¼ teaspoon cinnamon

Chocolate Sauce

2.5 ounces (70 g) 90% dark chocolate chips (85% or more), or sugar-free dark chocolate chips

1 tablespoon (15 ml) virgin coconut oil or cacao butter

INSTRUCTIONS

Prepare a batch of the Basic Sweet Chaffles by following the instructions on page 14, adding orange zest and cardamom. You can use a regular square 5-inch (12.5-cm) Belgian Waffle maker to make 2 chaffles or a mini waffle maker to make 3 chaffles. When the chaffles are done, let them cool down slightly, and then cut into a total of 8 (for square chaffles) or 9 (for mini chaffles) sticks.

Meanwhile, melt the dark chocolate with coconut oil and stir to combine. You can use a microwave oven or a double boiler. To use a double boiler, place a bowl over a saucepan filled with about 1 cup (240 ml) water. The bowl should not be touching the surface of the water. Bring to a boil and let it melt.

Serve the chaffle sticks with the chocolate sauce. The chaffle sticks can be stored just like Basic Sweet Chaffles (page 8).

Nutrition facts (2 chaffle sticks + about 1 tablespoon melted chocolate)

Total carbs:	Fiber:	Net carbs:	Protein:	Fat:	Calories:	Calories from
6.1 g	**1.8 g**	**4.3 g**	**8 g**	**20.6 g**	**228 kcal**	**carbs (7%)** **protein (14%)** **fat (79%)**

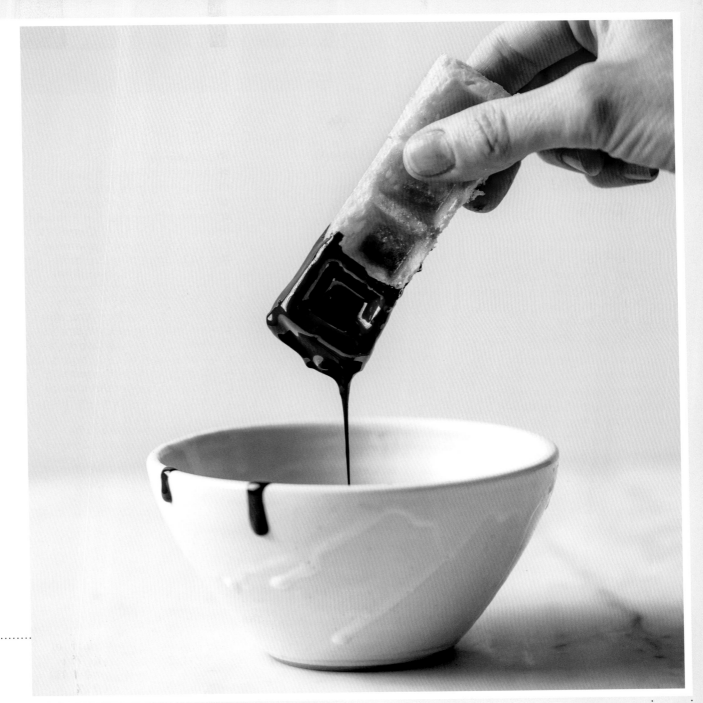

Apple Pie Chaffle Dippers

There is nothing as inviting as the smell of a freshly baked apple pie. I grew up eating loads of apple pies! At first, I was reluctant to try zucchini—it's a veggie, right? Let me tell you, even my neighbors weren't able to tell the difference. They thought I used apples! This apple butter has all of the amazing flavors of apple butter with a fraction of the carbs.

INGREDIENTS

Chaffles
Ingredients for Basic Sweet Chaffles (page 14)

½ teaspoon cinnamon

Apple Butter Dip
2 medium (500 g/1.1 lb.) zucchini, peeled (yields about 450 g/1 lb.)

¼ cup (57 g/2 oz) unsalted butter

2 tablespoons (30 ml) fresh lemon juice

½ cup (80 g/2.8 oz) brown sugar substitute, erythritol, or Swerve

1 teaspoon cinnamon, or to taste

⅛ teaspoon salt

Optional: serve with whipped cream, full-fat yogurt, or sour cream

Nutrition facts (2 chaffle sticks + about 2 tablespoons apple butter)

Total carbs:	Fiber:	Net carbs:	Protein:	Fat:	Calories:	Calories from
5 g	**1.5 g**	**3.5 g**	**7 g**	**13.2 g**	**161 kcal**	**carbs (9%) protein (17%) fat (74%)**

INSTRUCTIONS

Prepare a batch of the Basic Sweet Chaffles by following the instructions on page 14, adding cinnamon. You can use a regular square 5-inch (12.5-cm) Belgian Waffle maker to make 4 chaffles or a mini waffle maker to make 6 chaffles. Once the chaffles are done, let them cool down slightly, and then cut into a total of 16 (for square chaffles) to 18 (for mini chaffles) sticks.

Roughly chop the zucchini. Place it in a large saucepan with the butter, lemon juice, and sweetener. Bring to a simmer over medium-high heat, and then reduce the heat to medium-low. Cover and cook for 20 to 25 minutes, or until the zucchini begin to soften and fall apart. Remove from heat, allow to cool slightly, and use a hand blender to purée the mixture. Return the saucepan to medium-low heat. Add the cinnamon and salt. Gently simmer, stirring regularly to avoid spattering, until "apple" butter is thick and deep caramel in color, for 60 to 90 minutes. Transfer to a jar or sealed container.

Serve the sticks with the apple butter—warm or cold—and optionally with whipped cream, full-fat yogurt, or sour cream. Keep the apple butter refrigerated for up to 2 weeks. For longer storage freeze in an ice tray, and then empty the frozen apple butter cubes into a bag or container and store in the freezer for up to 6 months.

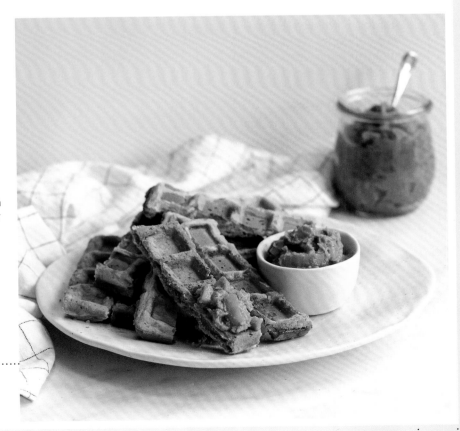

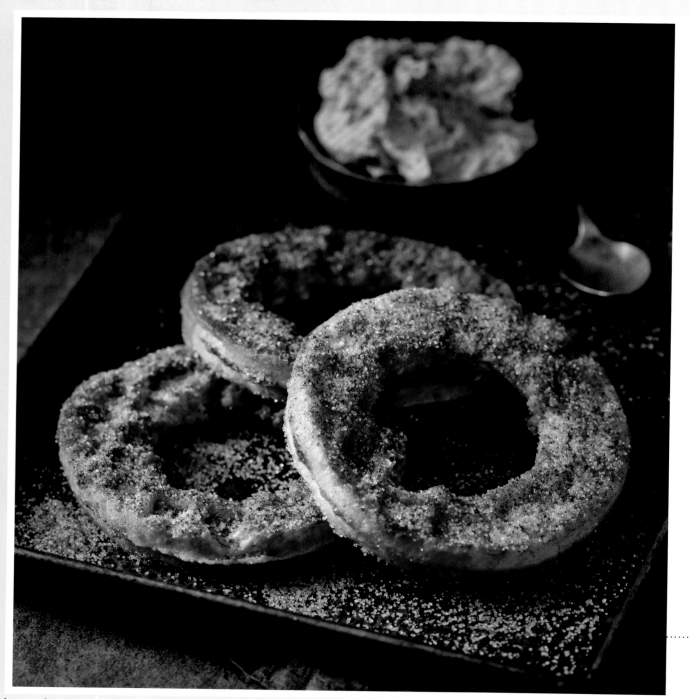

Servings:
**3 donuts +
donut holes**

Hands-on time:
15 minutes

Overall time:
20 minutes

Chaffle Donuts

This was an experimental recipe that went surprisingly well! Wonuts (waffle donuts) are nothing new, so why not try them with chaffles? They are first baked and then fried to get the flavor and crunch of real donuts! Serve with maple-flavored cream even your non-keto friends will love them.

INGREDIENTS

Donuts

3 Basic Sweet Chaffles (page 14)

2 tablespoons (20 g/0.7 oz) powdered low-carb sweetener such as erythritol or Swerve

1 teaspoon cinnamon

Coconut oil or ghee for frying

Maple Cream

⅔ cup (160 ml) heavy whipping cream

1 tablespoon (10 g/0.4 oz) powdered low-carb sweetener such as erythritol or Swerve

¼ teaspoon sugar-free maple extract or vanilla extract

INSTRUCTIONS

Prepare a batch of the Basic Sweet Chaffles by following the instructions on page 14.

While the chaffles are cooking, mix the erythritol with the cinnamon. Remove the chaffles from the waffle maker and while still warm, lightly dust with about half of the cinnamon-sweetener mixture (you can use a fine-mesh sieve or just a spoon). Use a 2.5-inch (6 cm) cookie cutter to cut out the center of each chaffle.

Heat a small saucepan or a frying pan filled with about ½ inch (1 cm) frying oil over medium-high heat. Fry the chaffles for just 30 seconds per side. Remove from the saucepan and dust with the remaining cinnamon-sweetener mixture. Use a fork to turn to the other side and dust more. Repeat the process for all the remaining chaffles, and, optionally, also the chaffle holes (or leave them plain).

In a small bowl whip the cream with sweetener and maple extract. Serve with the donuts and donut holes. Store any leftover cream in the fridge for up to 3 days. The donuts can be stored in a container covered with a kitchen towel for up to 3 days.

Nutrition facts (1 chaffle donut + 1 donut hole + about 4 tablespoons whipped cream)

Total carbs:	Fiber:	Net carbs:	Protein:	Fat:	Calories:	Calories from
5.9 g	**1.3 g**	**4.6 g**	**9.4 g**	**39 g**	**412 kcal**	**carbs (5%) protein (9%) fat (86%)**

Servings:
6 mini chaffles + about 300 g/ 10 oz ice cream

Hands-on time:
20 minutes

Overall time:
30 minutes + freezing

Chocolate Brownie Chaffles with Ice Cream

How does a warm slice of a soft brownie chaffle served with a scoop of creamy vanilla ice cream sound? Unlike brownies, these chaffles can be made in just a few minutes. And you won't need an ice cream maker to make perfectly fluffy ice cream!

INGREDIENTS

No-Churn Vanilla Ice Cream
2 large eggs, separated

⅛ teaspoon cream of tartar or apple cider vinegar

¼ cup (40 g/1.4 oz) powdered erythritol or Swerve

⅔ cup (160 ml) heavy whipping cream or coconut cream

1½ teaspoons sugar-free vanilla extract or ¾ teaspoon vanilla bean powder or a combination of the two

⅓ cup + 1 tablespoon (80 g/ 1.4 oz) granulated low-carb sweetener such as erythritol or Swerve

½ teaspoon gluten-free baking powder

1 teaspoon sugar-free vanilla extract

Optional: ¼ teaspoon instant coffee powder

Chaffles
2 large eggs

1 cup (113 g/4 oz) grated mozzarella

¼ cup (60 ml) melted butter or coconut oil

½ cup (50 g/1.8 oz) almond flour

¼ cup (22 g/0.8 oz) cacao powder or Dutch process cocoa powder

2 teaspoons (5 g/0.2 oz) flax meal or coconut flour

Chocolate Sauce
2.5 ounces (70 g) 90% dark chocolate chips (85% or more), or sugar-free dark chocolate chips

1 teaspoon virgin coconut oil or cacao butter

Nutrition facts (1 chaffle + 1 scoop ice cream + 2 teaspoons chocolate drizzle)

Total carbs:	Fiber:	Net carbs:	Protein:	Fat:	Calories:	Calories from
9.3 g	**3.1 g**	**6.2 g**	**13.1 g**	**37.3 g**	**412 kcal**	**carbs (6%) protein (13%) fat (81%)**

INSTRUCTIONS

To make the ice cream, whisk the egg whites with the cream of tartar in a large bowl. As the egg whites thicken, slowly add the powdered erythritol. Continue to whisk until stiff peaks form. In another bowl, whisk the cream until soft peaks form when the whisk is removed. (Be careful not to over-whisk the cream.) In a third bowl, mix the egg yolks with the vanilla. Slowly fold the whisked egg whites into the whipped cream. Then add the egg yolk mixture, and gently fold in with a spatula until well combined.

Place the mixture in a freezer-safe container. Freeze for at least 3 to 4 hours, or until set. For better portion control, divide the ice cream among three to six smaller containers. Let the ice cream sit at room temperature for 10 to 15 minutes before serving. Note: You will only need half a batch of the ice cream to serve with the chaffles (about 1 scoop/50 g/1.8 oz of fluffy ice cream per serving). Store the remaining ice cream in the freezer for up to 6 months.

While the ice cream is freezing, make the chaffles. Place all of the ingredients in a blender and process until smooth.

Spoon into a preheated mini waffle maker (about 62 g/2.2 oz per chaffle). Cook just like the Basic Sweet Chaffles (page 14). When the chaffles are done, let them cool down slightly.

Just before serving, melt the dark chocolate with coconut oil and stir to combine. You can use a microwave oven or a double boiler. To use a double boiler, place a bowl over a saucepan filled with about 1 cup (240 ml) water. The bowl should not be touching the surface of the water. Bring to a boil and let it melt.

Serve each chaffle with the vanilla ice cream and chocolate drizzle. The chaffles (no topping) can be stored just like Basic Chaffles (page 14).

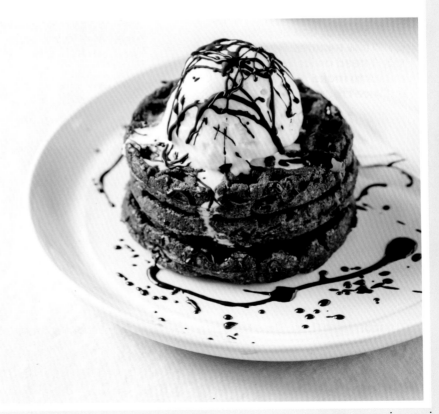

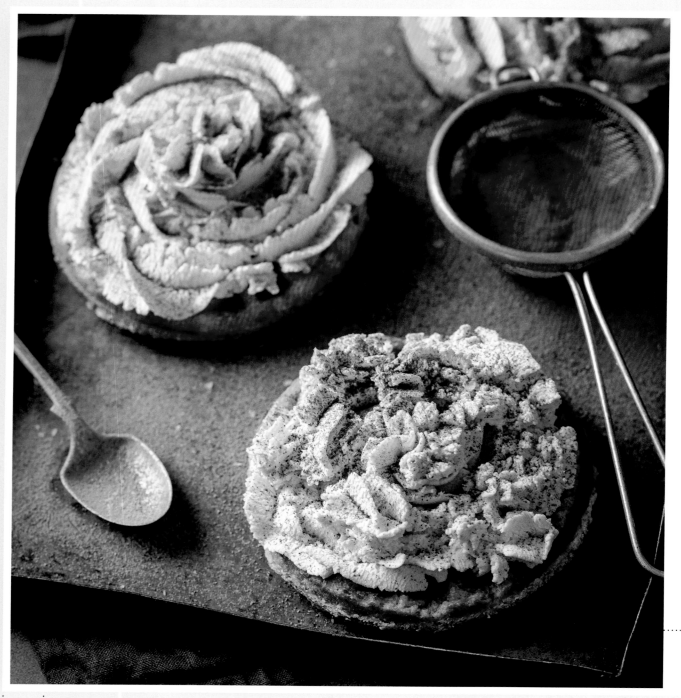

Sweet and Savory Keto Chaffles

Servings:
3 mini chaffles

Hands-on time:
10 minutes

Overall time:
15 minutes

Pumpkin-Spiced Latte Chaffles

This treat will remind you of that time of year when the weather gets cooler and pictures of pumpkin-spiced lattes start taking over social media. It is just like a cup of your favorite coffee in chaffle form!

INGREDIENTS

Chaffles

3 Basic Sweet Chaffles (page 14)

1 tablespoon (20 g/0.7 oz) pumpkin purée

2 teaspoons (6 g/0.2 oz) coconut flour

½ teaspoon pumpkin pie spice

Coffee Cream Topping

⅔ cup (160 ml) heavy whipping cream

1 tablespoon (10 g/0.4 oz) powdered low-carb sweetener such as erythritol or Swerve

1 teaspoon instant coffee or sugar-free coffee extract

Cinnamon for serving

INSTRUCTIONS

Prepare a batch of the Basic Sweet Chaffles by following the instructions on page 14, adding pumpkin purée, coconut flour, and pumpkin pie spice. When the chaffles are done, let them cool down slightly.

In a bowl, whip the cream with the sweetener and coffee. Pipe or spoon on top of each chaffle and dust with a pinch of cinnamon.

Decorated chaffles can be stored in a sealed jar in the fridge for 2 to 3 days.

Nutrition facts (1 chaffle + cream topping)

Total carbs:	Fiber:	Net carbs:	Protein:	Fat:	Calories:	Calories from
6.6 g	**1.6 g**	**5 g**	**9.9 g**	**30.3 g**	**338 kcal**	**carbs (6%)** **protein (12%)** **fat (82%)**

No-Tella Sandwich Chaffles

With this healthy version of the popular chocolate hazelnut spread, you won't be missing out on the real thing! I prefer this keto version because it's not super sweet and you can actually taste individual ingredients, not just sugar.

INGREDIENTS

No-Tella (makes about 450 g/1 lb.)

2¼ cups (300 g/10.4 oz) hazelnuts, peeled

1 bar (100 g/3.5 oz) 90% dark chocolate or chocolate chips (85% or more), or sugar-free dark chocolate

¼ cup (40 g/1.4 oz) powdered low-carb sweetener such as erythritol or Swerve, or to taste

1 tablespoon (6 g/0.2 oz) cacao powder

2 teaspoons (10 ml) sugar-free vanilla extract or ½ teaspoon vanilla powder

Optional: ⅛ teaspoon salt

Chaffles

4 Fluffy White Chaffles (Fluffy Sweet Chaffles Two Ways, page 90)

½ cup (120 g/4.2 oz) Keto No-Tella (recipe below)

2½ tablespoons (30 g/1.1 oz) 90% dark chocolate chips (85% or more), or sugar-free dark chocolate chips, melted

INSTRUCTIONS

Preheat the oven to 340°F (170°C) fan assisted or 375°F (190°C) conventional. Spread the hazelnuts on a baking tray and roast for 8 to 10 minutes, until slightly golden. Remove from the oven and allow to fully cool, about 15 minutes.

To melt the chocolate, place a bowl over a pan with boiling water and allow to melt, stirring occasionally. Once the nuts have cooled, add to a food processor and process until smooth. Add the sweetener, cacao powder, vanilla, salt (if using), and chocolate and pulse until combined. Pour the No-Tella into a jar and allow to cool and set in the fridge for 1 to 2 hours. The No-Tella can be stored in the fridge in a sealable jar for up to 3 months.

Prepare a batch of the Fluffy White Chaffles by following the instructions on page 91. When the No-Tella has set, spread a thick layer, about ¼ cup (60 g/ 2.1 oz), on top of two chaffles. Top each one with the remaining chaffles to make a total of 2 sandwiches. Press to seal and slice each sandwich in half to get a total of 4 servings. Drizzle with the melted chocolate, about 1 tablespoon (15 ml) for each chaffle sandwich.

Store in the fridge in a sealed container for up to 1 week.

Nutrition facts (½ chaffle sandwich + melted chocolate topping)

Total carbs:	Fiber:	Net carbs:	Protein:	Fat:	Calories:	Calories from
10.6 g	**4.3 g**	**6.3 g**	**12.8 g**	**30.1 g**	**344 kcal**	**carbs (7%) protein (15%) fat (78%)**

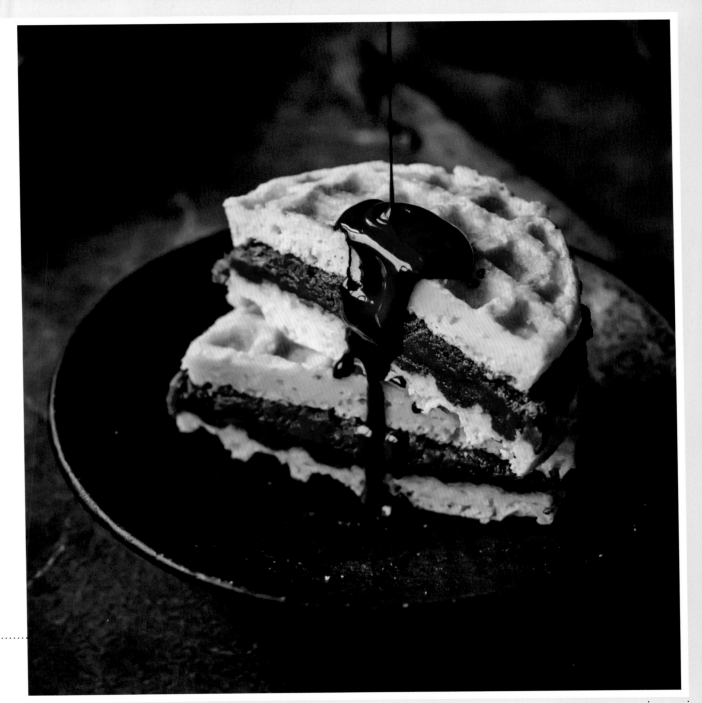

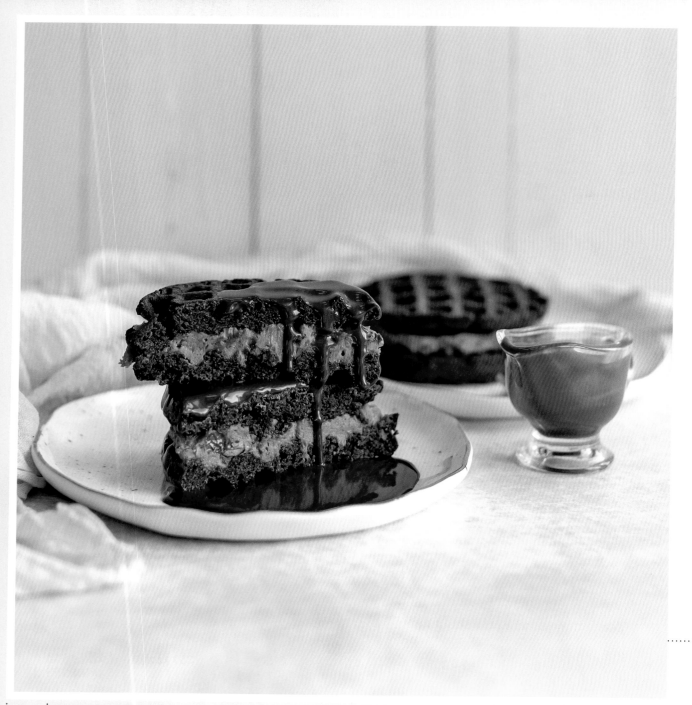

Servings:
2 chaffle sandwiches

Hands-on time:
15 minutes

Overall time:
20 minutes

Peanut Butter Cup Sandwich Chaffles

This recipe is for all peanut butter lovers. It's a super creamy peanut butter–cream layer served between two fluffy chocolate chaffles—what's not to love?

INGREDIENTS

Chaffles

4 Fluffy Chocolate Chaffles (Fluffy Sweet Chaffles Two Ways, page 90)

¼ cup (64 g/2.2 oz) roasted peanut butter or almond butter (smooth or chunky)

¼ cup (60 g/2.1 oz) mascarpone cheese

2 tablespoons (20 g/0.7 oz) powdered low-carb sweetener such as erythritol or Swerve, or to taste

Quick Ganache

¼ cup (60 ml) heavy whipping cream

3 tablespoons (35 g/1.2 oz) 90% dark chocolate chips (85% or more), or sugar-free dark chocolate chips

INSTRUCTIONS

Prepare a batch of the Fluffy Chocolate Chaffles by following the instructions on page 91. Let them cool down slightly. Place the peanut butter in a bowl with the mascarpone cheese and sweetener. Use a hand mixer to process until well combined. Spoon half of the mixture on top of two chaffles and top each with the remaining chaffle.

To make the quick chocolate ganache, heat the cream until hot and then pour it into a small bowl over the chocolate chips. Let it sit undisturbed for 1 to 2 minutes and then stir until smooth and glossy. Serve on top of the chaffles.

TIPS

* Instead of mascarpone cheese, you could use room-temperature unsalted butter. This will increase the calorie count too, so make sure to adjust for that.

* Instead of the chaffles used, you can make thinner chaffles (see page 91).

Nutrition facts (½ sandwich + about 1½ tablespoons chocolate ganache)

Total carbs:	Fiber:	Net carbs:	Protein:	Fat:	Calories:	Calories from
10 g	**3.2 g**	**6.8 g**	**13.8 g**	**31.3 g**	**359 kcal**	**carbs (7%) protein (15%) fat (78%)**

Servings:
2 chaffle stacks

Hands-on time:
20 minutes

Overall time:
25 minutes

Tiramisu Chaffles

I admit I do have a slight obsession with tiramisu, and I'm always on the look for new ways to make tiramisu-flavored treats. In these chaffles I kept the topping super simple, so you won't have to cook the egg yolks and whip up the egg whites like you would have to in a traditional tiramisu.

INGREDIENTS

4 Fluffy White Chaffles
(Fluffy Sweet Chaffles Two
Ways, page 90)

Coffee Liquid

3 tablespoons (45 ml) strong brewed coffee

1 tablespoon (15 ml) dark rum or 1½ teaspoons sugar-free rum extract

1 tablespoon (10 g/0.4 oz) powdered erythritol or Swerve, or a few drops of stevia

Cream Topping

⅓ cup (80 ml) heavy whipping cream

⅓ cup (80 g/2.8 oz) mascarpone

2 tablespoons (20 g/0.7 oz) powdered low-carb sweetener such as erythritol or Swerve, or to taste

¼ teaspoon sugar-free vanilla extract

2 teaspoons (4 g/0.2 oz) cacao powder or Dutch process cocoa, plus more for topping

INSTRUCTIONS

Prepare a batch of the Fluffy White Chaffles by following the instructions on page 91. Let them cool down slightly.

To make the coffee liquid, in a small bowl mix the coffee, rum, and sweetener. Place the 4 chaffles on a large plate and pour a tablespoon of the coffee liquid on each of the chaffles to soak.

In another bowl, mix the ingredients for the cream topping (use a whisk or ideally a mixer). Spoon the cream topping into a piping bag with a wide, round tip, and pipe small droplets onto each of the chaffles. If you want to keep it simple, use a spoon to spread the topping onto each chaffle. Dust with cacao powder and serve.

Tiramisu Chaffles can be stored in a sealed jar in the fridge for up to 5 days.

Nutrition facts (½ chaffle stack)

Total carbs:	Fiber:	Net carbs:	Protein:	Fat:	Calories:	Calories from
5.9 g	**1.7 g**	**4.2 g**	**10.1 g**	**24.8 g**	**292 kcal**	**carbs (6%)** **protein (14%)** **fat (80%)**

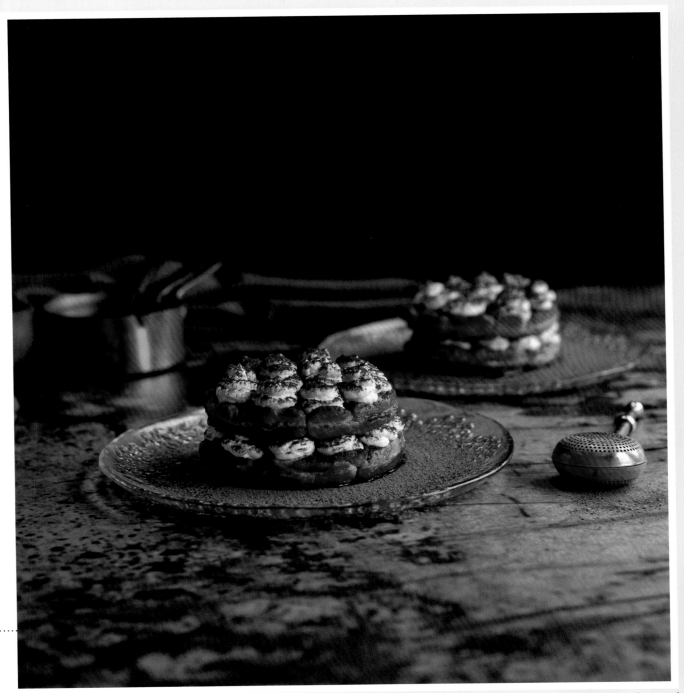

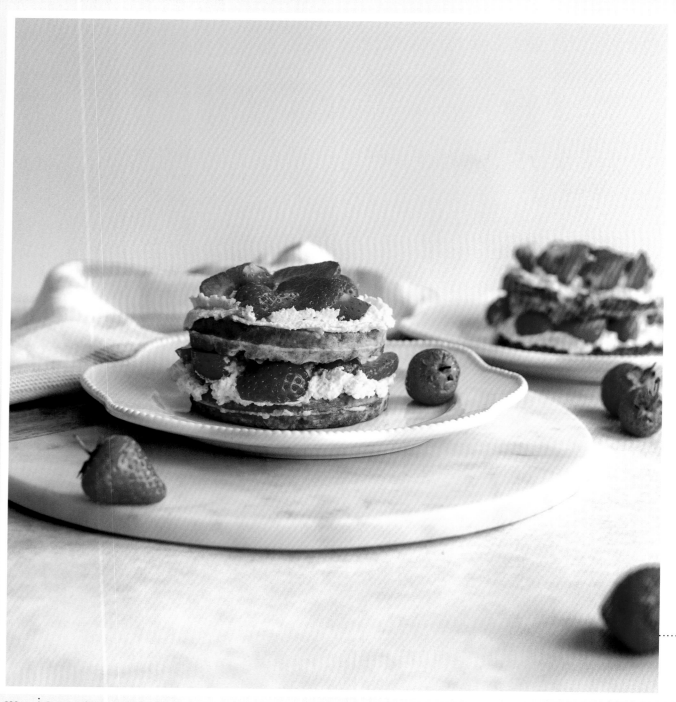

Servings:
2 chaffle stacks

Hands-on time:
10 minutes

Overall time:
15 minutes

Strawberry Shortcake Chaffles

These chaffles are like summer on a plate. They feature light and fluffy vanilla waffles with sweet fragrant strawberries. You won't even think about making a "real" strawberry shortcake!

INGREDIENTS

4 Fluffy White Chaffles (Fluffy Sweet Chaffles Two Ways, page 90)

1 cup (240 ml) heavy whipping cream

½ teaspoon sugar-free vanilla extract

Optional: 2 tablespoons (30 g/1.1 oz) powdered low-carb sweetener such as erythritol or Swerve, or to taste

4 large (80 g/2.8 oz) fresh strawberries, quartered, or berries of choice

INSTRUCTIONS

Prepare a batch of the Fluffy White Chaffles by following the instructions on page 91.

In a bowl, whip the cream with vanilla and optional sweetener. Top each chaffle with a quarter of the whipped cream and add a quarter of the strawberries. You can spoon on top or use a piping bag. Serve as single stacks or make chaffle sandwiches with more cream on top (½ stack per serving).

Decorated chaffles can be stored in a sealed jar in the fridge for 2 to 3 days.

Nutrition facts (½ chaffle stack)

Total carbs:	Fiber:	Net carbs:	Protein:	Fat:	Calories:	Calories from
7.2 g	**1.7 g**	**5.5 g**	**9.7 g**	**32.8 g**	**364 kcal**	**carbs (6%) protein (11%) fat (83%)**

White Chocolate Raspberry Mini Chaffle Cake

Easy, delicious, and so quick to prepare! This mini chaffle cake is filled with light and fluffy cream and topped with keto-friendly white chocolate drizzle. Everyone will adore this summer-inspired keto treat.

INGREDIENTS

3 Basic Sweet Chaffles (page 14)

Raspberry Cream Filling

⅔ cup (160 ml) heavy whipping cream

1 tablespoon (10 g/0.4 oz) powdered low-carb sweetener such as erythritol or Swerve, or to taste

⅛ teaspoon vanilla bean powder or ½ teaspoon sugar-free vanilla extract

⅔ cup (82 g/2.9 oz) fresh raspberries

White Chocolate Drizzle

1 tablespoon (16 g/0.6 oz) coconut butter (coconut manna)

1 tablespoon (14 g/0.5 oz) pieces of cacao butter or coconut oil

1 tablespoon (10 g/0.4 oz) powdered low-carb sweetener such as erythritol or Swerve, or to taste

⅛ teaspoon vanilla bean powder or ½ teaspoon sugar-free vanilla extract

Nutrition facts (⅓ mini chaffle cake)

Total carbs:	Fiber:	Net carbs:	Protein:	Fat:	Calories:	Calories from
9.4 g	**3.4 g**	**6 g**	**10 g**	**37.6 g**	**413 kcal**	**carbs (6%)** **protein (10%)** **fat (84%)**

INSTRUCTIONS

Prepare a batch of the Basic Sweet Chaffles by following the instructions on page 14.

To make the white chocolate topping, melt the coconut butter with cacao butter in a microwave. Stir in the powdered sweetener and vanilla.

In a bowl, whip the cream with vanilla and optional sweetener. Fold in the raspberries (optionally leave a few for topping). You can spoon the cream on top or use a piping bag.

To assemble, make a stack of 3 chaffles (⅓ stack per serving), or top each chaffle with one-third of the cream and drizzle each with about 1 tablespoon (15 ml) of the white chocolate topping.

Decorated chaffles can be stored in a sealed jar in the fridge for 2 to 3 days.

TIPS

✻ Instead of 3 Basic Sweet Chaffles (serves 3), you can use 4 Fluffy White Chaffles (Fluffy Sweet Chaffles Two Ways, page 90) to make 4 servings (2 chaffle sandwiches cut in half). You can also triple the recipe and make four large round 7-inch (18-cm) Belgian waffles to make a regular-sized cake (12 servings).

✻ If you can get proper keto-friendly white chocolate, feel free to swap for the topping. Instead of the vanilla in the white chocolate drizzle, you can use ½ teaspoon freshly grated lemon zest.

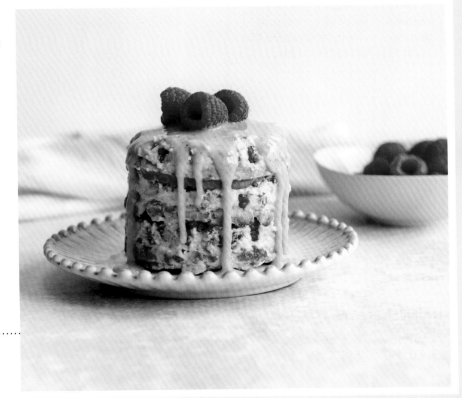

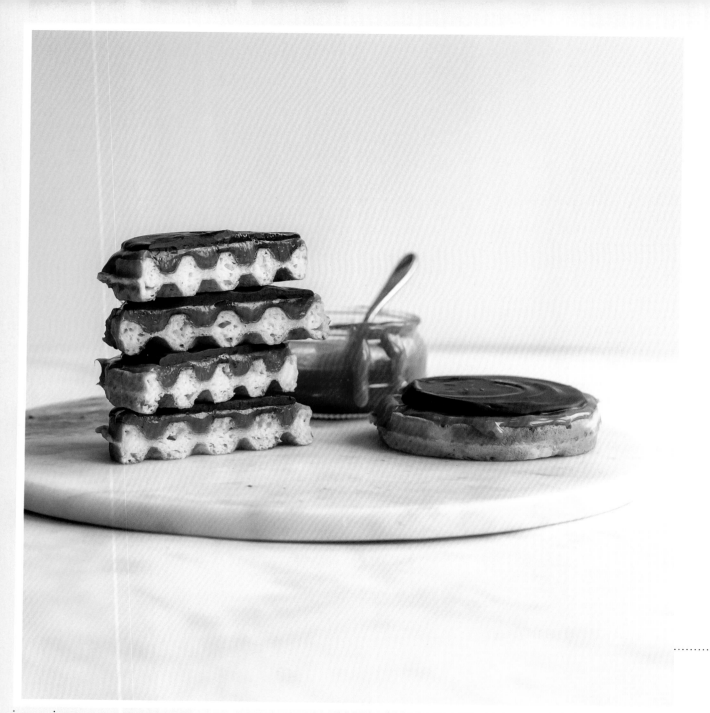

Servings:
3 mini chaffles

Hands-on time:
15 minutes

Overall time:
20 minutes

Millionaire's Shortbread Chaffles

What if I told you that caramel was not off limits? This chaffle is all you ever wish for in a caramel treat. It's smooth and creamy salted caramel served on a shortbread chaffle. You will never know it's keto!

INGREDIENTS

Chaffles
1 large egg

½ cup (57 g/2 oz) grated mozzarella

½ cup (50 g/1.8 oz) more almond flour

1½ tablespoons (15 g/0.5 oz) powdered low-carb sweetener such as erythritol or Swerve

¼ teaspoons gluten-free baking powder

Chocolate Topping
2.5 ounces (70 g) 90% dark chocolate chips (85% or more), or sugar-free dark chocolate chips

1 teaspoon virgin coconut oil

Caramel Filing
6 tablespoons (90 g/3.2 oz) chilled Keto Caramel (page 11)

INSTRUCTIONS

To make the caramel, follow steps on page 11. This will take an extra hour to prepare.

To prepare the chaffles, preheat a mini waffle maker and follow the instructions for the Basic Sweet Chaffles (page 14) but with the ingredients listed in this recipe. Each chaffle will be made from about 57 g/2 oz of the batter. When the chaffles are done, let them cool down completely.

Meanwhile, melt the dark chocolate with coconut oil and stir to combine. You can use a microwave oven or a double boiler (see page 109 for instructions). Let it cool down to room temperature.

Spread 2 tablespoons (30 g/1.1 oz) of the cooled caramel on top of each chaffle. Spoon the melted chocolate topping on top and let it set for a few minutes before serving. Slice in half and enjoy immediately, or store at room temperature in a container covered with a kitchen towel for up to 1 day, in the fridge for up to 1 week, or freeze for up to 3 months.

Nutrition facts (½ chaffle)

Total carbs:	Fiber:	Net carbs:	Protein:	Fat:	Calories:	Calories from
5.6 g	**1.6 g**	**4 g**	**6.4 g**	**21.3 g**	**229 kcal**	**carbs (7%)** **protein (11%)** **fat (82%)**

Servings:
4 chaffle stacks

Hands-on time:
15 minutes

Overall time:
20 minutes

Banoffee Chaffles

These chaffles are super easy with a fraction of the carbs in a traditional banoffee pie. With no condensed milk, no bananas, and only 100% keto caramel, this British-inspired dessert will make your taste buds sing!

INGREDIENTS

4 Fluffy Chocolate Chaffles (page 90; you'll make 8 super thin chaffles)

¼ cup (60 g/2.1 oz) chilled Keto Caramel (page 11)

1¼ cups (300 ml) heavy whipping cream

3 tablespoons (30 g/1.1 oz) powdered low-carb sweetener such as erythritol or Swerve, or to taste

1 to 2 teaspoons sugar-free banana extract

2 small squares (10 g/0.4 oz) 90% dark chocolate (85% or more) or sugar-free dark chocolate

INSTRUCTIONS

To make the caramel, follow steps on page 11. This will take an extra 30 minutes to 1 hour to prepare.

To make the chaffles, follow the recipe on page 90, but make 8 super thin chaffles instead of 4. Each of the chaffles will be made from about 31 g/1.1 oz of the batter (2 level tablespoons). Make sure to cook them for just 30 to 60 seconds as they burn easily. If you prefer to make 4 regular chaffles, you can carefully cut them widthwise while they are still warm.

Whip the cream with sweetener and banana extract. Spread 1 tablespoon (15 g/0.5 oz) of the caramel on top of 4 thin chaffles. Spoon or pipe half of the whipped cream on top of the 4 chaffles. Top each with the remaining chaffles and add the remaining whipped cream. Grate dark chocolate over the chaffle sandwiches and serve or store them in a sealed container the fridge for up to 4 days.

Nutrition facts (1 chaffle stack)

Total carbs:	Fiber:	Net carbs:	Protein:	Fat:	Calories:	Calories from
8.4 g	**1.9 g**	**6.5 g**	**9.5 g**	**43.9 g**	**465 kcal**	**carbs (6%)** **protein (8%)** **fat (86%)**

TIP

✳ If you can handle a few extra carbs, feel free to swap the banana extract for a few slices of banana. Remember, carbs are not evil and contrary to a common myth, you don't have to avoid all whole foods that contain carbs. Low-carb and keto eating is not about removing all carbs but finding the level of carbohydrate that works best for your unique needs.

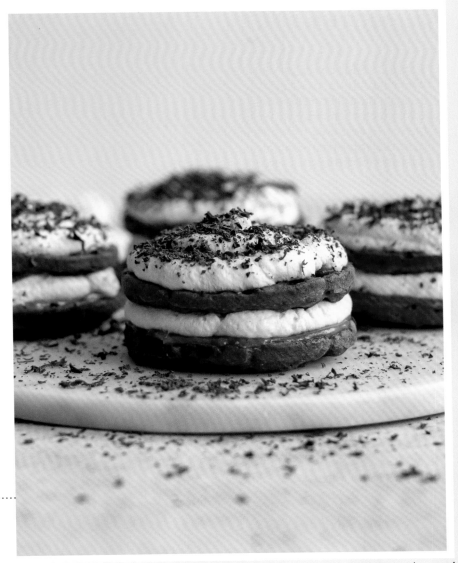

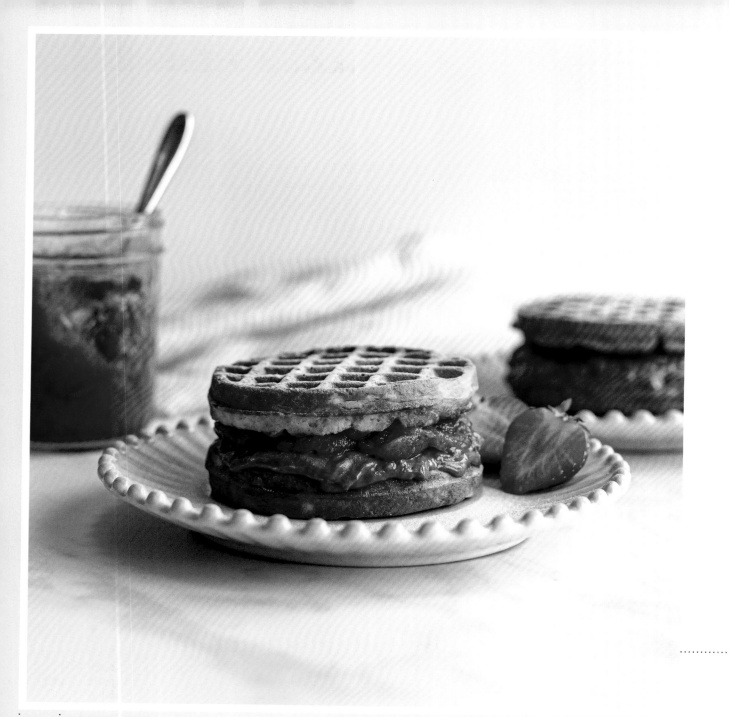

Sweet and Savory Keto Chaffles

Servings:
2 chaffle sandwiches

Hands-on time:
20 minutes

Overall time:
1 hour

PB & J Sandwich Chaffles

If you want to take the notoriously popular peanut butter & jelly to the next level, make these keto-friendly chaffle sandwiches. They look pretty and they are easy to make, easy to pack, and easy to eat!

INGREDIENTS

Strawberry Jelly (makes about 370 g/13 oz)

1½ teaspoons (6 g/0.2 oz) gelatin powder

12 ounces (340 g) fresh or frozen and thawed strawberries

1 tablespoon (15 ml) fresh lemon or lime juice

3 tablespoons (30 g/1.1 oz) powdered low-carb sweetener such as erythritol or Swerve, or to taste

Chaffles

4 Fluffy White Chaffles (Fluffy Sweet Chaffles Two Ways, page 90)

¼ cup (64 g/2.2 oz) roasted peanut butter or almond butter (smooth or chunky)

¼ cup (60 g/2.1 oz) Strawberry Jelly (recipe below)

Optional: powdered erythritol or Swerve

INSTRUCTIONS

To make the strawberry jelly, place the gelatin to a small bowl filled with 2 tablespoons (30 ml) water. Leave to bloom for a few minutes. Place the strawberries in a blender and pulse until smooth.

Place half of the blended strawberries in a saucepan. Heat over medium-low heat and add the bloomed gelatin. Cook briefly and stir until melted. Remove from the heat and add the lemon juice, sweetener, and the rest of the strawberries. Place in a jar and allow to cool. Once cool, transfer to the fridge for about 30 minutes or up to 1 hour to set. If you like more of a set jam, use as is. If you prefer a softer jam, give the jam a really good stir until it loosens up and is smooth. Store in a sealed glass jar in the fridge.

To make the chaffles, follow the recipe for Fluffy White Chaffles on page 90. Let them cool down completely. Top two chaffles with peanut butter (half each), followed by the set strawberry jelly (half each). Top each with the remaining chaffles and lightly press in. Optionally, dust with powdered low-carb sweetener and slice.

Serve immediately or store in a sealed jar in the fridge for up to 4 days.

Nutrition facts (½ chaffle sandwich)

Total carbs:	Fiber:	Net carbs:	Protein:	Fat:	Calories:	Calories from
8.1 g	**2.5 g**	**5.6 g**	**12.8 g**	**18.3 g**	**232 kcal**	**carbs (9%) protein (22%) fat (69%)**

Servings:
3 chaffle sandwiches

Hands-on time:
15 minutes

Overall time:
20 minutes

Fudgy Chocolate Sandwich Chaffles

This recipe is for all chocolate lovers! Rich and decadent chocolate buttercream filling is piped between two thin and light chocolate waffles. Feel free to add whipped cream on top!

INGREDIENTS

Chaffles
4 Fluffy Chocolate Chaffles (page 90; you'll make 6 thinner chaffles)

Chocolate Buttercream Filling
½ cup (125 g/4.4 oz) coconut butter (coconut manna) or smooth almond butter, softened

¼ cup (60 ml) melted virgin coconut oil

½ cup (113 g/4 oz) unsalted butter, room temperature

3 tablespoons (16 g/0.6 oz) cacao powder or Dutch process cocoa powder

3 tablespoons (30 g/1.1 oz) powdered low-carb sweetener such as erythritol or Swerve, or to taste

INSTRUCTIONS

Prepare a batch of the Fluffy Chocolate Chaffles by following the instructions on page 91, but make 6 thinner chaffles instead of 4 regular thickness (see tip on page 91). Let them cool down slightly.

To make the buttercream filling, place all of the ingredients into a bowl and use a hand mixer to process until smooth and creamy. Spoon the chocolate buttercream into a piping bag and top 3 out of the 6 chaffles, or simply spoon on top. Top with the remaining chaffles and gently press in.

Cut in half and enjoy immediately, or store in a sealed container in the fridge for up to 5 days.

Nutrition facts (½ chaffle sandwich)

Total carbs:	Fiber:	Net carbs:	Protein:	Fat:	Calories:	Calories from
9.2 g	**5.3 g**	**3.9 g**	**6.9 g**	**33.2 g**	**344 kcal**	**carbs (5%)** **protein (8%)** **fat (87%)**

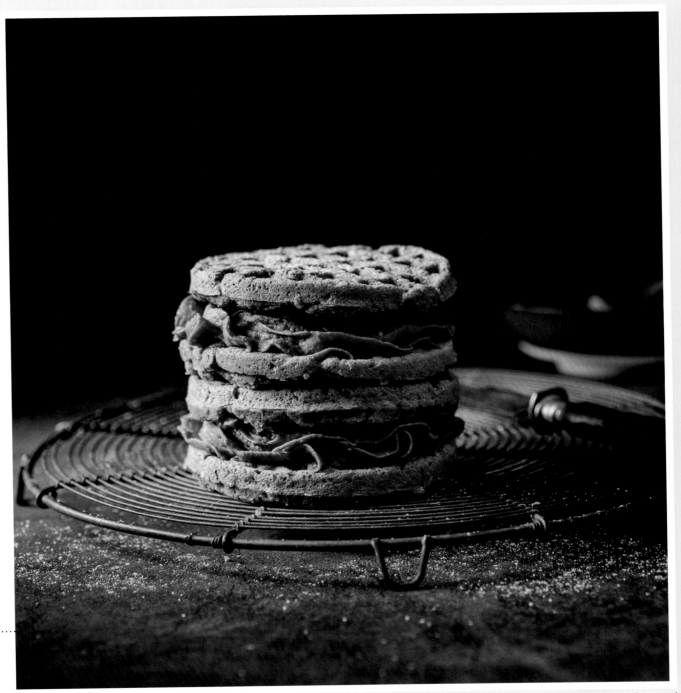

Servings:
8 s'mores sandwiches

Hands-on time:
30 minutes

Overall time:
1 hour

S'mores Chaffles

Did you know you can make perfectly fluffy marshmallows that can be toasted and taste like the real deal? Once you know how to make sugar-free marshmallows you're just a step away from making the most delicious chaffle S'mores!

INGREDIENTS

Marshmallows (makes 16 large marshmallows)
2 tablespoons (22 g/0.8 oz) gelatin powder

⅔ cup (133 g/4.7 oz) allulose, or to taste (see tip)

1 teaspoon sugar-free vanilla extract

⅛ teaspoon salt

Chaffles
6 Basic Sweet Chaffles (page 14, you'll make 4 square chaffles)

8 large squares (80 g/2.8 oz) 90% dark chocolate (85% or more) or sugar-free dark chocolate

8 Keto Marshmallows (recipe at right)

INSTRUCTIONS

Line a baking dish with parchment paper or use a silicon baking dish. Sprinkle the gelatin in a cup filled with ⅓ cup (80 ml) of water and let the gelatin bloom (soak up the liquid) for a few minutes.

Meanwhile, make simple syrup by heating ½ cup (120 ml) of water with allulose. Stir and heat up over medium heat until boiling and fully dissolved. Shake and tilt if needed to dissolve fully. Cook for 2 to 3 minutes. If you've got a thermometer it should reach about 210°F (100°C).

You'll have to work quickly to make sure the syrup is still hot. For the next step you should ideally use a stand mixer. You could use a hand mixer, but keep in mind you'll need to hold it for 15 minutes! Place the bloomed gelatin into your stand mixer and turn on low to break up the bloomed gelatin. Quickly pour in the hot syrup straight on the gelatin, not on the sides of the mixing bowl so it retains the heat when it touches the gelatin. Increase the speed to high and whisk for about 10 minutes. Sprinkle in the salt about halfway through, and the vanilla just a minute or two before it's done.

Nutrition facts (1 chaffle S'more)

Total carbs:	Fiber:	Net carbs:	Protein:	Fat:	Calories:	Calories from
5.3 g	**1.3 g**	**4 g**	**8.4 g**	**12.9 g**	**163 kcal**	**carbs (10%) protein (20%) fat (70%)**

When ready, the mixture will be fluffy and stiff. Turn the mixer off and quickly spread the marshmallow in a lined dish or a silicon dish. You'll need to work fast as it may solidify. Let the marshmallows dry uncovered at room temperature overnight. Remove from the baking dish (10 × 10 inch/25 × 25 cm) and cut with a greased knife into 16 pieces. You'll only need 8 marshmallows. Store the leftover 8 marshmallows in a cool dry place for about 1 week.

To make the chaffles, follow the instructions for the Basic Sweet Chaffles on page 14, but use a square 5-inch Belgian waffle maker instead of round mini waffle maker to make a total of 2 regular-sized (5-inch/12.5-cm) Belgian square chaffles. Let them cool slightly and then use a sharp knife to cut each in quarters.

To assemble the S'mores, place a square (10 g/0.4 oz) of dark chocolate on top of each chaffle quarter and top with the marshmallow piece. Use a blow torch to melt (or place under a broiler for a few seconds) and then top with the remaining chaffle quarters.

These are best eaten freshly made, but they can be stored at room temperature for up to 1 day.

TIP

✱ I like using allulose as this natural low-carb sweetener does not crystalize once chilled. It's also perfect for the smoothest keto caramel, page 11! If you can't find allulose, use erythritol or Swerve. Feel free to adjust the level of sweetness by using a few tablespoons less or more sweetener.

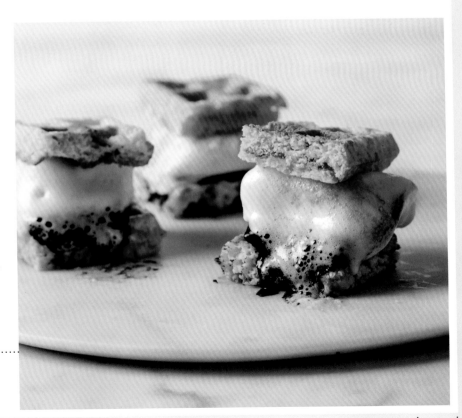

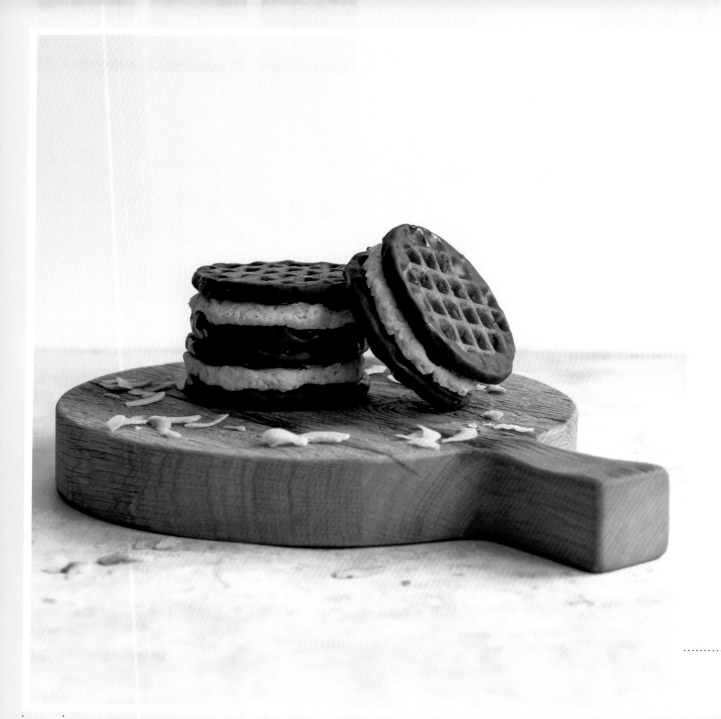

Servings:
3 chaffle sandwiches

Hands-on time:
15 minutes

Overall time:
25 minutes

Paradise Bar Chaffles

These chaffles—two thin layers of chocolate chaffles with a delicious toasted coconut surprise—taste like your favorite candy bars!

INGREDIENTS

Chaffles

4 Fluffy Chocolate Chaffles (Fluffy Sweet Chaffles Two Ways, page 90; you'll make 6 thin chaffles)

Coconut Filling

½ cup (38 g/1.3 oz) unsweetened shredded coconut

3 tablespoons (30 g/1.1 oz) powdered low-carb sweetener such as erythritol or Swerve, or to taste

½ teaspoon sugar-free vanilla extract

¼ cup (45 g/1.6 oz) coconut cream

2 teaspoons (10 ml) virgin coconut oil

Chocolate Crust

2.5 ounces (70 g) 90% dark chocolate chips (85% or more), or sugar-free dark chocolate chips

1 teaspoon virgin coconut oil

INSTRUCTIONS

Prepare a batch of the Fluffy Chocolate Chaffles by following the instructions on page 91, but make 6 thinner chaffles (see tip on page 91). Let them cool down slightly.

Preheat the oven to 350°F (175°C) fan assisted or 380°F (195°C, or gas mark 5) conventional. Place the coconut on a baking tray and bake in the preheated oven for 5 to 6 minutes. Remove from the oven and let cool down for 10 minutes. Mix the toasted coconut, sweetener, vanilla, coconut cream, and coconut oil.

Meanwhile, melt the dark chocolate with coconut oil and stir to combine. You can use a microwave oven or a double boiler (see page 109 for instructions). Let it cool down to room temperature. Dip the edges of each of the chaffle in the chocolate slowly turning the chaffle as you coat it to create a chocolate rim all around. Drizzle any leftover chocolate on top.

Spoon about 2½ tablespoons (41 g/1.5 oz) of the coconut mixture onto 3 chaffles and top with the remaining chaffles to create 3 sandwiches. Gently press down and slice to serve or place in a sealed container and store in the fridge for up to 1 week.

Nutrition facts (½ chaffle sandwich)

Total carbs:	Fiber:	Net carbs:	Protein:	Fat:	Calories:	Calories from
7.6 g	**3.1 g**	**4.5 g**	**7.7 g**	**16.9 g**	**204 kcal**	**carbs (9%) protein (15%) fat (76%)**

Servings:
3 chaffle sandwiches

Hands-on time:
15 minutes

Overall time:
20 minutes

Cannoli Chaffles

Nothing beats the combination of crunchy, dark chocolate–crusted chaffles filled with the creamiest ricotta orange-flavored cream. They're classic Italian cream-filled pastries made low-carb!

INGREDIENTS

Chaffles
Ingredients for 4 Fluffy White Chaffles (page 90, you'll make 6 thinner chaffles)

¼ teaspoon cinnamon

Ricotta Orange Filling
¾ cup (180 g/6.4 oz) ricotta cheese, drained

3 tablespoons (30 g/1.1 oz) powdered low-carb sweetener such as erythritol or Swerve, or to taste

1 teaspoon fresh orange zest

1 teaspoon sugar-free vanilla extract

Chocolate Crust & Coating
2.5 ounces (70 g) 90% dark chocolate chips (85% or more), or sugar-free dark chocolate chips

1 teaspoon virgin coconut oil

3 tablespoons (20 g/0.7 oz) slivered almonds

INSTRUCTIONS

Prepare a batch of the Fluffy White Chaffles by following the instructions on page 91, adding cinnamon to the batter. Make 6 thinner chaffles instead of 4 regular thickness (see tip on page 91). Let them cool down slightly.

To make the filling, in a bowl beat the ricotta, sweetener, orange zest, and vanilla with a balloon whisk or a spatula.

Meanwhile, melt the dark chocolate with coconut oil and stir to combine. You can use a microwave oven or a double boiler (see page 109 for instructions). Let it cool down to room temperature. Dip the edges of each of the chaffle in the chocolate slowly turning the chaffle as you coat it to create a chocolate rim all around. Drizzle any leftover chocolate on top.

Spoon about ⅓ cup (about 72 g/2.5 oz) of the cream mixture onto 3 chaffles and top with the remaining chaffles to create 3 sandwiches.

Roll the sides in slivered almonds and serve, or place in a sealed container and store in the fridge for up to 3 days. These will be crispy when freshly made and hard to slice so either cut them in half before filling or refrigerate and slice the next day.

Nutrition facts (½ chaffle sandwich)

Total carbs:	Fiber:	Net carbs:	Protein:	Fat:	Calories:	Calories from
7.1 g	**2.1 g**	**5 g**	**10.9 g**	**19.7 g**	**240 kcal**	**carbs (8%)** **protein (18%)** **fat (74%)**

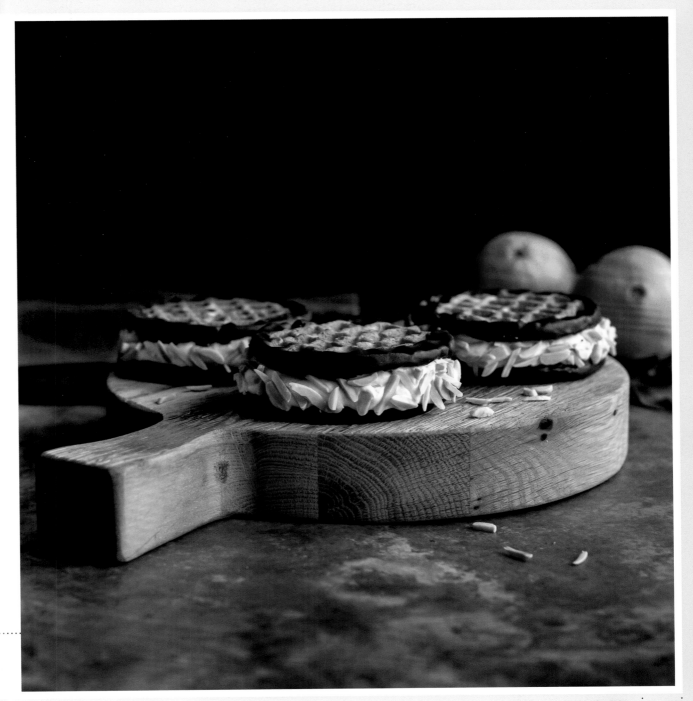

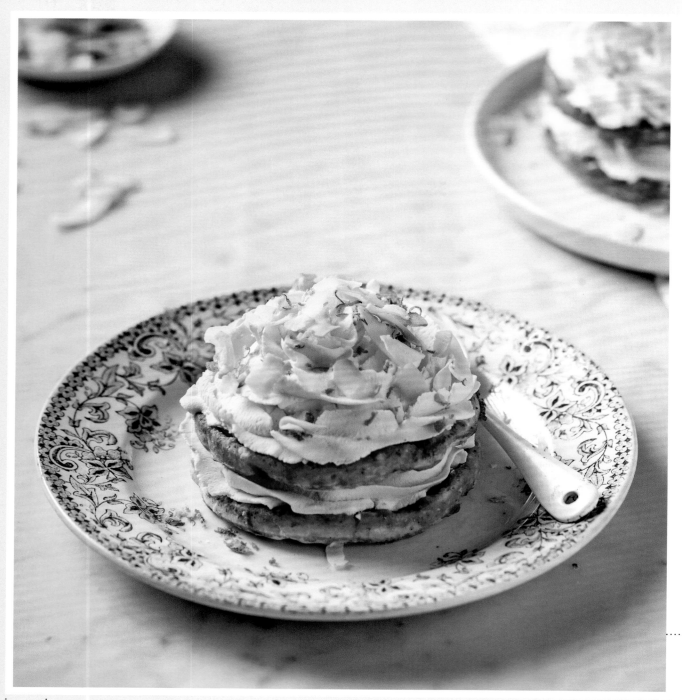

Sweet and Savory Keto Chaffles

Servings:
3 chaffle stacks

Hands-on time:
15 minutes

Overall time:
20 minutes

Coconut & Lime Cheesecake Chaffles

If you're the kind of person who likes to enjoy a dessert for breakfast, this lime-flavored cheesecake chaffle topped with toasted coconut won't disappoint. And if you're throwing a dinner party, this tropical treat will look so cute!

INGREDIENTS

Topping

¼ cup (15 g/0.5 oz) unsweetened coconut chips

Optional: lime or lemon zest

Chaffles

4 Fluffy White Chaffles (page 90; you'll make 6 thinner chaffles)

Cheesecake Filling

¾ cup (180 ml) heavy whipping cream

½ cup (120 g/4.2 oz) cream cheese or mascarpone

½ teaspoon fresh lime zest, plus more to taste

3 tablespoons (30 g/1.1 oz) powdered low-carb sweetener such as erythritol or Swerve, or to taste

1 tablespoon (15 ml) fresh lime juice

INSTRUCTIONS

Place the coconut chips in a hot, dry pan and roast for a minute or two, until lightly browned and crispy. Once crisped up, slide into a bowl and let them cool down.

Prepare a batch of the Fluffy White Chaffles by following the instructions on page 91, adding cinnamon to the batter. Make 6 thinner chaffles instead of 4 of regular thickness (see tip on page 91). Let them cool down slightly.

To make the cheesecake filling, use a whisk or ideally a mixer to combine the whipping cream, cream cheese, lime zest, sweetener, and lime juice. Spoon the cream topping into a piping bag for pretty cheesecake roses. If you want to keep it simple, use a spoon to spread the topping onto each chaffle.

Sprinkle with the toasted coconut chips and optionally with more lime zest. These chaffles can be stored in a sealed jar in the fridge for up to 5 days.

Nutrition facts (½ chaffle stack)

Total carbs:	Fiber:	Net carbs:	Protein:	Fat:	Calories:	Calories from
5.2 g	**1.3 g**	**3.9 g**	**7.7 g**	**25.3 g**	**268 kcal**	**carbs (6%) protein (11%) fat (83%)**

Servings:
6 eclairs

Hands-on time:
30 minutes

Overall time:
1 hour + chilling

Chocolate Chaffle Eclairs

Say hi to the best keto eclairs! Using waffles instead of the traditional choux pastry works surprisingly well in this creamy custard pastry. Plus it's easy to double the batch because you'll have plenty of crème pâtissière to do that!

INGREDIENTS

Crème Pâtissière (makes about 620 g/1.4 lb.)

½ teaspoon gelatin powder

½ cup (120 ml) heavy whipping cream

1½ cups (360 ml) unsweetened almond milk

6 large egg yolks

½ cup + 2½ tablespoons (85 g/2.8 oz) granulated low-carb sweetener such as erythritol or Swerve, or to taste

1 tablespoon sugar-free vanilla extract or about 1 teaspoon vanilla powder

Pinch of salt

½ cup (113 g/4 oz) unsalted butter, chopped into 6 to 8 pieces

Chaffles

4 Fluffy White Chaffles (page 90; you'll make 3 square chaffles)

¾ cup (180 g/6.4 oz) Crème Pâtissière

Chocolate Ganache

3 tablespoons (45 ml) heavy whipping cream

⅓ cup (57 g/2 oz) 90% dark chocolate chips (85% or more), or sugar-free dark chocolate chips

1½ tablespoons (21 g/0.7 oz) unsalted butter

Nutrition facts (1 eclair)

Total carbs:	Fiber:	Net carbs:	Protein:	Fat:	Calories:	Calories from
5.6 g	**1.6 g**	**4 g**	**7.8 g**	**26 g**	**280 kcal**	**carbs (6%)** **protein (11%)** **fat (83%)**

INSTRUCTIONS

To make the crème pâtissière, sprinkle the gelatin in a small bowl filled with 1 tablespoon (15 ml) water and set aside.

In a medium saucepan, heat the heavy whipping cream and almond milk over medium-high heat. While it's heating, place the egg yolks in a bowl with the sweetener, vanilla, and salt. Using a hand mixer or a balloon whisk, beat until smooth and frothy.

Once the milk starts boiling and foam starts to form, take it off the heat. Use a ladle to gradually temper the hot mixture into the egg mixture. Keep whisking constantly or the mixture will curdle. When the eggs have been tempered, add the egg mixture back into the hot milk in the saucepan. Whisk vigorously and cook over medium heat until it starts to thicken, about 2 minutes. Cook for 3 to 4 minutes. Take it off the heat and add the bloomed gelatin, and then stir in the butter. Pour the mixture into a container and let it cool down to room temperature. You can speed up the chilling by placing the container in ice water and stirring occasionally until cool. Cover with a lid and refrigerate overnight.

To make the chaffles, follow the instructions for the Basic Chaffles on page 14, but use a square 5-inch (12.5-cm)

Belgian waffle maker instead of round mini waffle maker to make a total of 3 regular-sized (5-inch/12.5 cm) Belgian square chaffles. While they are still warm, use a sharp knife to cut each chaffle in half and then cut each half widthwise to create a total of 12 thinner waffle slices (2 per eclair).

To make the ganache, heat the cream until hot and then pour in a small bowl over the chocolate chips and butter. Let it sit undisturbed for 1 to 2 minutes, and then stir until smooth and glossy. Set aside.

Spoon about 2 tablespoons (30 g/ 1.1 oz) of crème pâtissière into a piping bag and pipe on the cut side of 6 chaffle pieces. Top with the remaining 6 chaffles and then drizzle each one with the

chocolate ganache. Let the ganache set for a few minutes. Serve immediately or store in a sealed container for up to 4 days.

TIP

* If you want to use vanilla beans or vanilla powder instead, add the seeds or the powder to the saucepan with the hot cream and almond milk. Stain through a fine-mesh sieve before adding to the egg mixture.

* Apart from making eclairs, use any leftover crème pâtissière as topping for berries or simply to spread on any sweet chaffles.

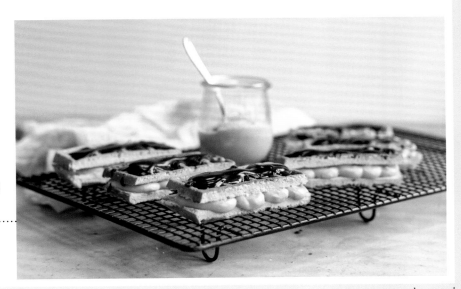

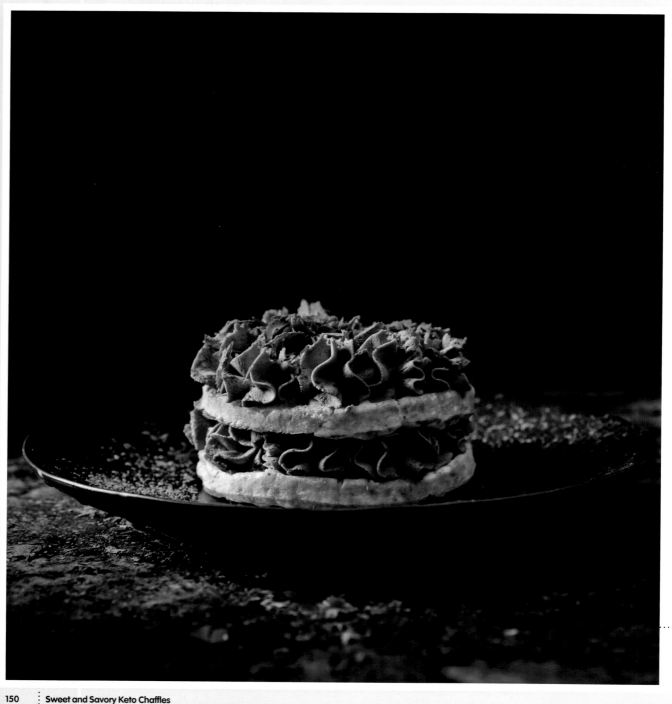

Chocolate Cheesecake Chaffles

Delicious layers of chocolate cheesecake piped onto light and fluffy chaffles. If you want to enhance the chocolate flavor, add a pinch of cinnamon and coffee powder and you've got the ultimate chocolate treat!

INGREDIENTS

Chaffles
4 Fluffy White Chaffles (page 90; you'll make 6 thinner chaffles)

2 small squares (10 g/0.4 oz) 90% dark chocolate or sugar-free dark chocolate, grated; or use chocolate shavings

Optional: pinch of cinnamon or cacao powder

Cheesecake Filling
¾ cup (180 ml) heavy whipping cream

½ cup (120 g/4.2 oz) cream cheese or mascarpone

¼ cup (40 g/1.4 oz) powdered low-carb sweetener such as erythritol or Swerve, or to taste

3 tablespoons (16 g/0.6 oz) cacao powder or Dutch process cocoa powder

½ teaspoon sugar-free vanilla extract

¼ teaspoon cinnamon

Optional: ¼ to ½ teaspoon instant coffee powder

Optional: dark chocolate shavings

INSTRUCTIONS

Prepare a batch of the Fluffy White Chaffles by following the instructions on page 91. Make 6 thinner chaffles instead of 4 regular thickness (see tip on page 91). Let them cool down slightly.

To make the cheesecake filling, use a whisk or ideally a mixer to mix the whipping cream, cream cheese, sweetener, cacao powder, vanilla, cinnamon, and optionally coffee powder. Spoon the cream topping into a piping bag for pretty cheesecake roses. If you want to keep it simple, use a spoon to spread the topping onto each chaffle. Top with grated chocolate or chocolate shavings. Dust with more cinnamon or cacao powder, or sprinkle with dark chocolate shavings. These chaffles can be stored in a sealed jar in the fridge for up to 5 days.

TIP

* To make chocolate shavings, melt the dark chocolate and spread a thin later on a slab of marble or a small plate. Place in the fridge to set for 1 to 2 minutes and then just make thin flakes by scraping it off.

Nutrition facts (½ chaffle stack)

Total carbs:	Fiber:	Net carbs:	Protein:	Fat:	Calories:	Calories from
6.5 g	**2.1 g**	**4.4 g**	**8.3 g**	**25 g**	**268 kcal**	**carbs (6%) protein (12%) fat (82%)**

Servings:
1 cake (12 slices)

Hands-on time:
30 minutes

Overall time:
1 hour

Triple Chocolate Chaffle Cake

Making a decadent chocolate cake that will impress everyone has never been easier. This luscious keto chocolate cake made with layers of chaffles and fluffy chocolate cream is ideal for family gatherings and celebrations, or for when you just feel like enjoying a slice a cake!

INGREDIENTS

Chaffles (triple batch of Fluffy Chocolate Chaffles, page 90)

3 large eggs

3 large egg whites

⅓ cup + 1 tablespoon (90 g/3.2 oz) cream cheese

1½ cups (170 g/6 oz) grated mozzarella

6 tablespoons (33 g/1.2 oz) cacao powder

6 tablespoons (48 g/1.7 oz) coconut flour

½ cup + 2 tablespoons (120 g/4.2 oz) granulated low-carb sweetener such as erythritol or Swerve

1½ teaspoons gluten-free baking powder

Chocolate Filling

1⅔ cups (400 ml) heavy whipping cream

⅓ cup (53 g/1.9 oz) powdered low-carb sweetener such as erythritol or Swerve

⅓ cup (29 g/1 oz) cacao powder or Dutch process cocoa powder

1 tablespoon (15 ml) sugar-free vanilla extract

Chocolate Ganache

½ cup (85 g/3 oz) 90% dark chocolate chips (85% or more), or sugar-free dark chocolate chips

¼ cup (60 ml) heavy whipping cream

2 tablespoons (28 g/1 oz) unsalted butter

Nutrition facts (1 slice, ¹⁄₁₂ cake chaffle cake)

Total carbs:	Fiber:	Net carbs:	Protein:	Fat:	Calories:	Calories from
8.6 g	**3.1 g**	**5.5 g**	**9.5 g**	**28.1 g**	**314 kcal**	**carbs (7%)** **protein (12%)** **fat (81%)**

INSTRUCTIONS

Prepare a batch of the Fluffy Chocolate Chaffles by following the instructions on page 91, but instead make 3 chaffles or 4 thinner 7-inch (18-cm) round chaffles (see tip on page 91). Let them cool down completely.

Meanwhile, make the chocolate filling. Whip the cream with the sweetener, cacao powder, and vanilla until fluffy and stiff (do not overbeat).

To assemble the cake, spread part of the whipped cream filling on top of one chaffle. Add another chaffle and lightly press in. Repeat until all of the chaffles are used, finishing with the last layer of whipped chocolate cream. Spread the remaining cream on the sides of the cake. Place in the fridge to set for 30 to 60 minutes.

To make the ganache, heat the cream until hot and then pour into a small bowl over the chocolate chips and butter. Let it sit undisturbed for 1 to 2 minutes and then stir until smooth and glossy. Pour the ganache over the top of the cake and the sides.

Slice and serve, or store in the fridge for up to 5 days.

TIP

* If a whole cake is too much for you, only make one batch (4 mini waffles) of the Fluffy Chocolate Chaffles, a third of the chocolate cream filling, and a third of the ganache to make 1 mini cake made with 4 mini chaffles (¼ cake per serving).

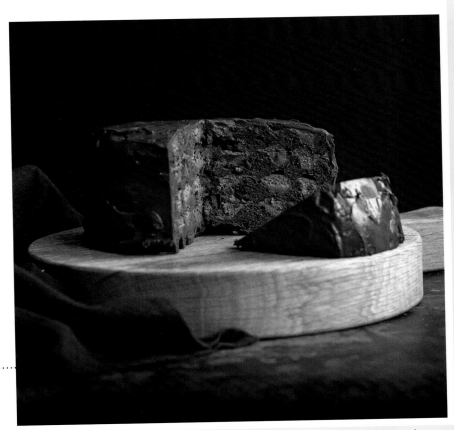

Servings:
1 cake (12 slices)

Hands-on time:
30 minutes

Overall time:
1 hour

Birthday Chaffle Cake

Want to make an easy—yet impressive—birthday treat for that special someone? This is pretty much the easiest way to make cake, so make sure to involve the kids! Feel free to decorate with berries or swap the sugar-free confetti for dark chocolate chips to make a cake for any special occasion.

INGREDIENTS

Chaffles (triple batch of Fluffy White Chaffles, page 90)

3 large eggs

3 large egg whites

⅓ cup + 1 tablespoon (90 g/3.2 oz) cream cheese

1½ cups (170 g/6 oz) grated mozzarella

¾ cup (75 g/2.7 oz) almond flour

½ cup + 2 tablespoons (120 g/4.2 oz) granulated low-carb sweetener such as erythritol or Swerve

1½ teaspoons gluten-free baking powder

2 teaspoons (10 ml) sugar-free vanilla extract or ½ teaspoon vanilla powder

3 tablespoons (42 g/1.5 oz) sugar-free confetti (see tips)

Buttercream Frosting

2½ sticks (283 g/10 oz) unsalted butter, room temperature

Small pinch of salt

2 cups (160 g/5.6 oz) powdered low-carb sweetener such as erythritol or Swerve

1 tablespoon (15 ml) sugar-free vanilla extract

¼ cups (60 ml) heavy whipping cream

¼ cup (58 g/2 oz) sour cream or more heavy whipping cream

3 tablespoons (42 g/1.5 oz) sugar-free confetti to topping, or to taste

Nutrition facts (1 slice, ¹/₁₂ cake chaffle cake)

Total carbs:	Fiber:	Net carbs:	Protein:	Fat:	Calories:	Calories from
6.2 g	**1.3 g**	**4.9 g**	**8.8 g**	**31.9 g**	**342 kcal**	**carbs (6%)** **protein (10%)** **fat (84%)**

INSTRUCTIONS

Prepare a batch of the Fluffy White Chaffles by following the instructions on page 91, but instead make 3 chaffles or up to 4 thinner 7-inch (18-cm) round chaffles (see tip on page 91). Stir in the confetti just before you bake the chaffles or sprinkle them on top as you spoon the batter into the waffle maker. Let them cool down completely.

Meanwhile, make the buttercream frosting. Place the butter in the bowl of your stand mixer or use a hand mixer to beat it on medium-high speed for 5 to 6 minutes. This is important as it will make the butter fluffy. Add the salt and slowly add the sweetener until well combined. Add the vanilla, cream, and sour cream, and beat on low speed until combined and fluffy.

To assemble the cake, put about a quarter of the buttercream (about 155 g/ 5.5 oz) on top of one chaffle. Add another chaffle and lightly press in. Repeat until all of the chaffles are used, finishing with the third layer of buttercream, and then spread the remaining buttercream around the sides.

Decorate with more confetti. Slice and serve, or refrigerate for up to 4 days. This is best served at room temperature so let it sit at room temperature for about 30 minutes before serving. For longer storage, freeze for up to 3 months.

TIPS

∗ You can find sugar-free confetti in some online stores, but they are only available in some countries. If you can't get sugar-free confetti, either skip them or swap them for dark chocolate chips to make a chocolate chip cookie cake instead.

∗ Just like your typical birthday cake, this chaffle cake is very sweet, even though I used a fraction of the amount of sweetener that is typically used in frosting. Feel free to adjust the sweetener to your liking or use lightly sweetened whipped cream instead of the buttercream.

∗ If a whole cake is too much for you, only make one batch (4 mini waffles) of the Fluffy White Chaffles and a third of the buttercream filling to make 1 mini cake made with 4 mini chaffles (¼ cake per serving).

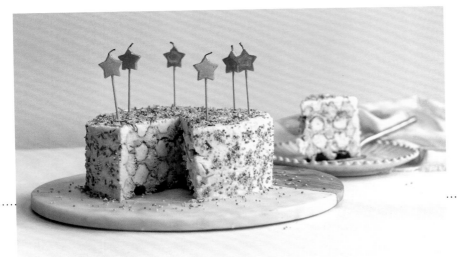

About the Author

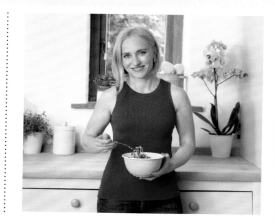

Martina Slajerova is a health and food blogger living in the United Kingdom. She holds a degree in economics and worked in auditing but has always been passionate about nutrition and healthy living. Martina loves food, science, and photography, and she enjoys creating new recipes. She is a firm believer in low-carb living and regular exercise. As a science geek, she bases her views on valid research and has firsthand experience of what it means to be on a low-carb diet. Both are reflected on her blog, in her KetoDiet apps, and in this book.

The KetoDiet is an ongoing project she started with her partner in 2012 and includes *The KetoDiet Cookbook, Sweet and Savory Fat Bombs, Quick Keto Meals in 30 Minutes or Less, Keto Slow Cooker & One-Pot Meals, The Beginner's KetoDiet Cookbook, The Keto All Day Cookbook, Keto Simple,* and the KetoDiet apps for iOS (iPad, iPhone, and Android [www.ketodietapp.com]). When creating recipes, she doesn't focus solely on the carb content: You won't find any processed foods, unhealthy vegetable oils, or artificial sweeteners in her recipes.

This book and the KetoDiet apps are for those who follow a healthy, low-carb lifestyle. Martina's mission is to help you reach your goals, whether that means reaching your dream weight or simply eating healthy food. You can find even more low-carb recipes, diet plans, expert guides, and information about the keto diet on her blog: www.ketodietapp.com/blog.

Acknowledgments

I'd like to thank the amazing team at Fair Winds Press, who put so much hard work into my cookbooks. It's been an absolute pleasure working with you! Special thanks to Jill Alexander, Renae Haines, Heather Godin, Jenna Patton, and Todd Conly.

Index